THE POCKET DOCTOR

Obstetrics and Gynecology

THE POCKET DOCTOR

Obstetrics and Gynecology

Richa Saxena MBBS, MD
Obstetrician and Gynecologist
New Delhi, India

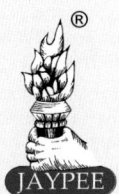

JAYPEE BROTHERS MEDICAL PUBLISHERS (P) LTD
New Delhi • London • Philadelphia • Panama

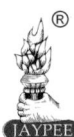
Jaypee Brothers Medical Publishers (P) Ltd

Headquarters

Jaypee Brothers Medical Publishers (P) Ltd
4838/24, Ansari Road, Daryaganj
New Delhi 110 002, India
Phone: +91-11-43574357
Fax: +91-11-43574314
Email: jaypee@jaypeebrothers.com

Overseas Offices

J.P. Medical Ltd
83 Victoria Street, London
SW1H 0HW (UK)
Phone: +44-2031708910
Fax: +02-03-0086180
Email: info@jpmedpub.com

Jaypee-Highlights Medical Publishers Inc.
City of Knowledge, Bld. 237, Clayton
Panama City, Panama
Phone: + 507-301-0496
Fax: + 507-301-0499
Email: cservice@jphmedical.com

Jaypee Medical Inc.
The Bourse
111 South Independence Mall East
Suite 835, Philadelphia, PA 19106, USA
Phone: + 267-519-9789
Email: jpmed.us@gmail.com

Jaypee Brothers Medical Publishers (P) Ltd
17/1-B Babar Road, Block-B, Shaymali
Mohammadpur, Dhaka-1207
Bangladesh
Mobile: +08801912003485
Email: jaypeedhaka@gmail.com

Jaypee Brothers Medical Publishers (P) Ltd
Bhotahity, Kathmandu, Nepal
Phone: +977-9741283608
Email: kathmandu@jaypeebrothers.com

Website: www.jaypeebrothers.com
Website: www.jaypeedigital.com

© 2014, Jaypee Brothers Medical Publishers

The views and opinions expressed in this book are solely those of the original contributor(s)/author(s) and do not necessarily represent those of editor(s) of the book.

All rights reserved. No part of this publication may be reproduced, stored or transmitted in any form or by any means, electronic, mechanical, photocopying, recording or otherwise, without the prior permission in writing of the publishers.

All brand names and product names used in this book are trade names, service marks, trademarks or registered trademarks of their respective owners. The publisher is not associated with any product or vendor mentioned in this book.

Medical knowledge and practice change constantly. This book is designed to provide accurate, authoritative information about the subject matter in question. However, readers are advised to check the most current information available on procedures included and check information from the manufacturer of each product to be administered, to verify the recommended dose, formula, method and duration of administration, adverse effects and contraindications. It is the responsibility of the practitioner to take all appropriate safety precautions. Neither the publisher nor the author(s)/editor(s) assume any liability for any injury and/or damage to persons or property arising from or related to use of material in this book.

This book is sold on the understanding that the publisher is not engaged in providing professional medical services. If such advice or services are required, the services of a competent medical professional should be sought.

Every effort has been made where necessary to contact holders of copyright to obtain permission to reproduce copyright material. If any have been inadvertently overlooked, the publisher will be pleased to make the necessary arrangements at the first opportunity.

Inquiries for bulk sales may be solicited at: jaypee@jaypeebrothers.com

The Pocket Doctor: Obstetrics and Gynecology

First Edition: **2014**

ISBN : 978-93-5090-701-6

Printed at : Samrat Offset Pvt. Ltd.

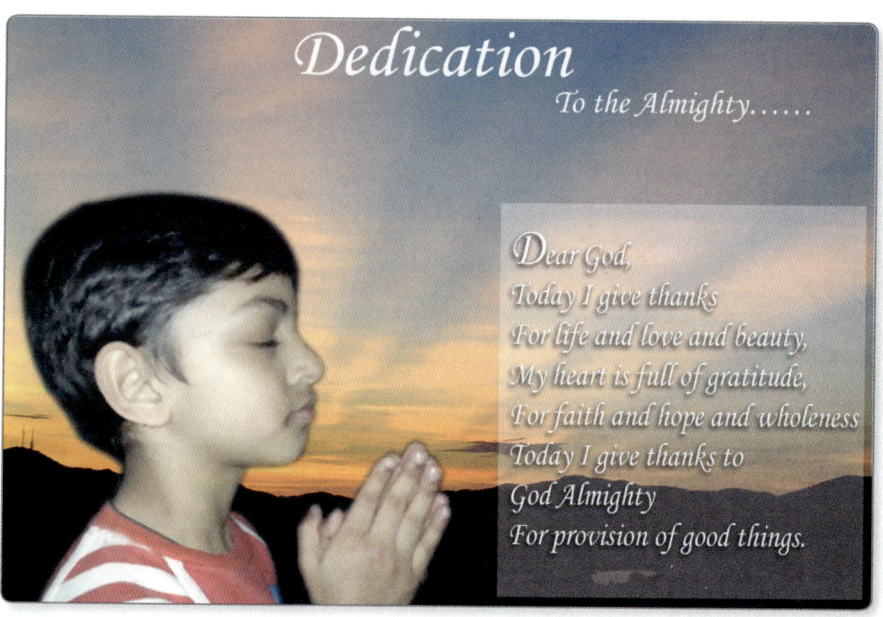

PREFACE

This book on obstetrics and gynecology belonging to the Jaypee's "The Pocket Doctor" serves as a compilation of nearly 150 evidence-based protocols, which would prove extremely useful for the practicing clinicians in this era of evidence-based medicine. This book holds a series of step-by-step, well-elucidated, standardized, well-agreed, evidence-based protocols, which would be of extreme help to the clinicians. The book would help in complementing the textbooks on obstetrics and gynecology and aid the busy clinician in developing an organized, condensed and practical approach towards patient care. The text is thoroughly updated and is given in a style, which is easy-to-understand and grasp, without having to go through elaborate text. The Flow Charts have been liberally illustrated with help of colored photographs and illustrations wherever required. In order to ensure that a Flow Chart is able to provide complete information on its own, pinned-up color boxes have also been added in the Flow Charts. They contain matter relevant to that provided by the Flow Chart. In order to ensure that each chapter contains all the information in a concise manner, tables have also been provided along with the Flow Charts and pictures. Following these protocols while delivering patient care would serve as a catalyst towards improvement of overall standard of medical care and in ensuring uniform patient care. The book would serve as a ready reckoner and a good source of reference carrying snippets of useful information for residents and practitioners in obstetrics and gynecology as well as general practitioners.

Richa Saxena

CONTENTS

PART 1 OBSTETRICS

Section 1 Management in Antenatal Period

Chapter 1 Surveillance in the Antenatal Period	2
Chapter 2 Smoking and Drug Abuse During Pregnancy	5
Chapter 3 Common Pregnancy-Related Problems	7

Section 2 Abnormal Presentation

Chapter 4 Breech Presentation	16
Chapter 5 Transverse Lie	19

Section 3 Pregnancy-Related Complications

Chapter 6 Antepartum Hemorrhage	24
Chapter 7 Twin Pregnancy	35
Chapter 8 Rh-Negative Pregnancy	39
Chapter 9 Hydatidiform Mole	47
Chapter 10 Fetal Growth Restriction	52
Chapter 11 Preterm Pregnancy	56
Chapter 12 Post-Term Pregnancy	58
Chapter 13 Polyhydramnios	60
Chapter 14 Urogenital Fistula Due to Obstructed Labor	63
Chapter 15 Miscarriage	65
Chapter 16 Previous Cesarean Section	70

Section 4 Medical Complications During Pregnancy

Chapter 17 Preeclampsia	76
Chapter 18 Gestational Diabetes	81
Chapter 19 Anemia in Pregnancy	86
Chapter 20 Heart Disease During Pregnancy	90
Chapter 21 Asthma During Pregnancy	92
Chapter 22 Thyroid Disorders During Pregnancy	94
Chapter 23 Malaria in Pregnancy	99
Chapter 24 Pregnancy in Obese Women	100

Section 5   Postnatal Period

Chapter 25   Postpartum Hemorrhage 104
Chapter 26   Amniotic Fluid Embolism 109

PART 2   GYNECOLOGY

Section 6   General

Chapter 27   Normal Gynecological Examination 112

Section 7   Abnormalities in Menstruation

Chapter 28   Abnormal Uterine Bleeding Due to Endometrial Cancer 116
Chapter 29   Dysfunctional Uterine Bleeding 122

Section 8   Benign Masses

Chapter 30   Leiomyomas 126

Section 9   Infections in Pregnancy

Chapter 31   Vaginal Discharge 132

Section 10   Malignancies of the Genital Tract

Chapter 32   Cervical Cancer 136
Chapter 33   Ovarian Neoplasms 139

Section 11   Pain

Chapter 34   Pelvic Pain 144
Chapter 35   Ectopic Pregnancy 148
Chapter 36   Dysmenorrhea 151

Section 12   Abnormalities in Conception

Chapter 37   Infertility 154
Chapter 38   Amenorrhea 158
Chapter 39   Polycystic Ovarian Syndrome 163
Chapter 40   Hirsutism 166

Abbreviations *171*

OBSTETRICS

Section 1

Management in Antenatal Period

- **Chapter 1** Surveillance in the Antenatal Period
- **Chapter 2** Smoking and Drug Abuse During Pregnancy
- **Chapter 3** Common Pregnancy-Related Problems

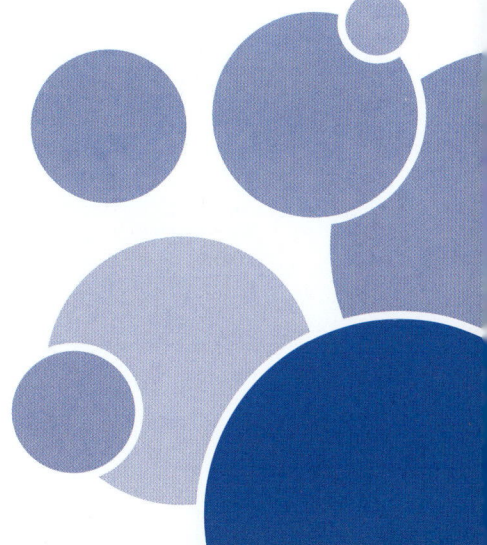

1 Surveillance in the Antenatal Period

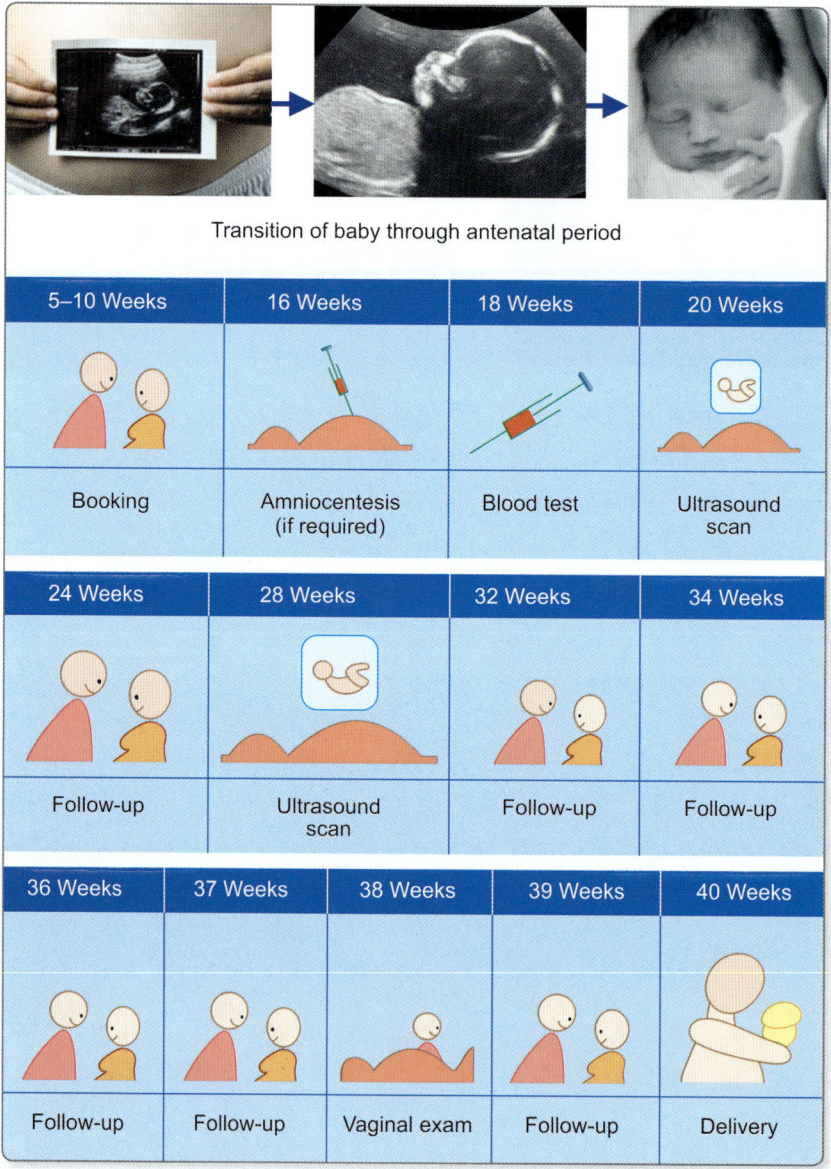

Transition of baby through antenatal period

5–10 Weeks	16 Weeks	18 Weeks	20 Weeks
Booking	Amniocentesis (if required)	Blood test	Ultrasound scan

24 Weeks	28 Weeks	32 Weeks	34 Weeks
Follow-up	Ultrasound scan	Follow-up	Follow-up

36 Weeks	37 Weeks	38 Weeks	39 Weeks	40 Weeks
Follow-up	Follow-up	Vaginal exam	Follow-up	Delivery

Antenatal Schedule

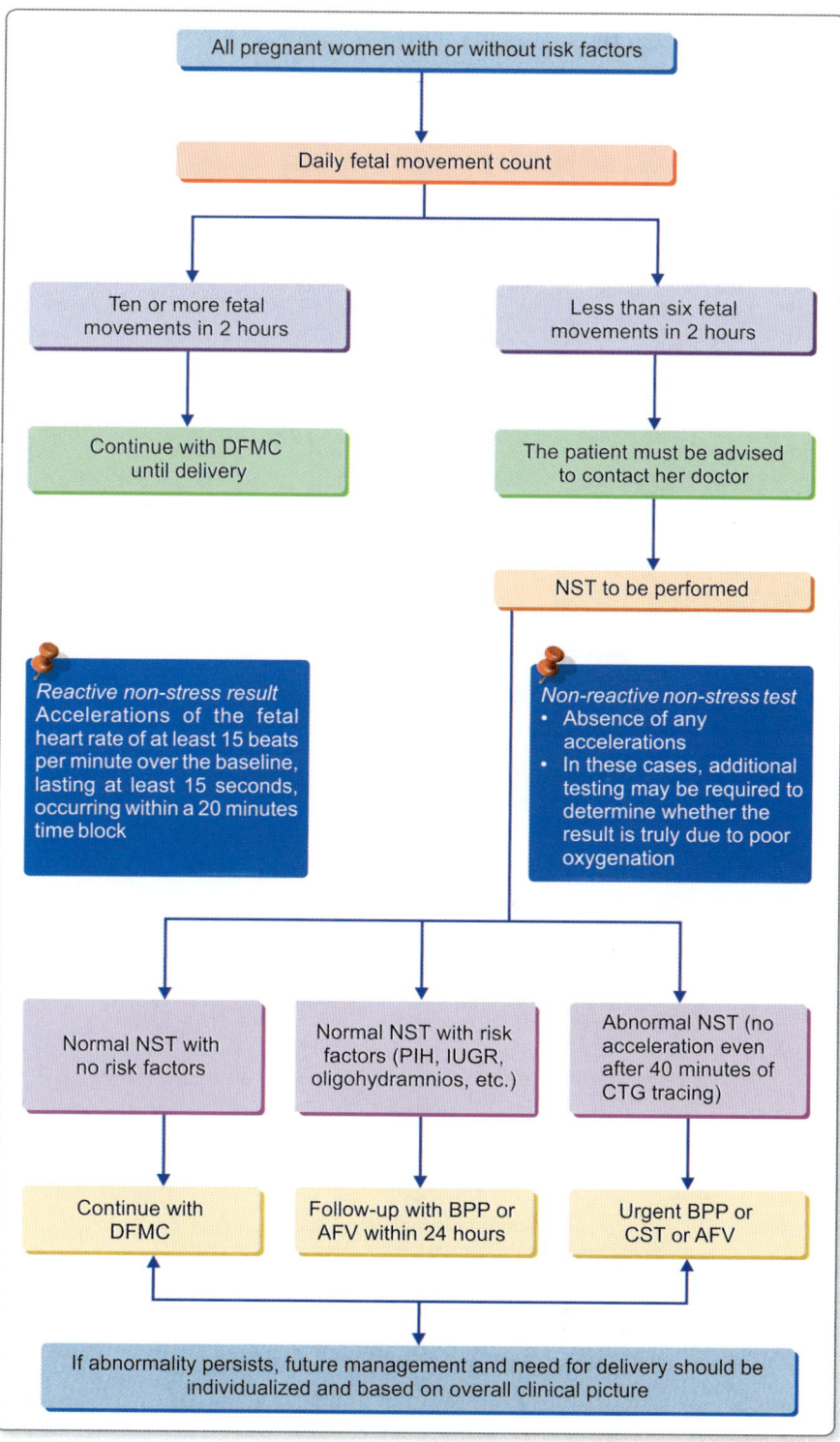

Flow Chart 1.1   Management protocol for antepartum fetal surveillance

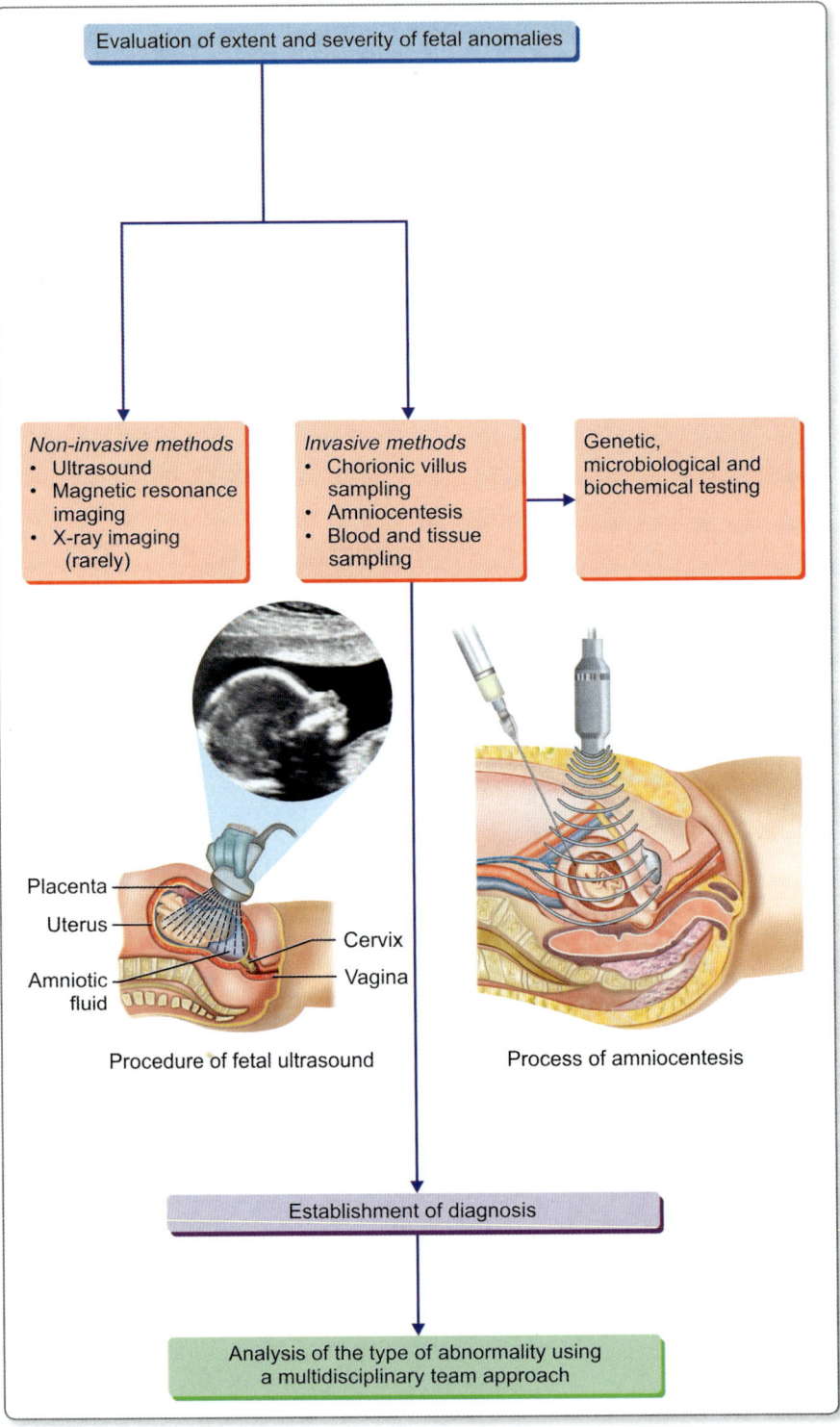

Flow Chart 1.2 Prenatal diagnosis of fetal anomalies

2 Smoking and Drug Abuse During Pregnancy

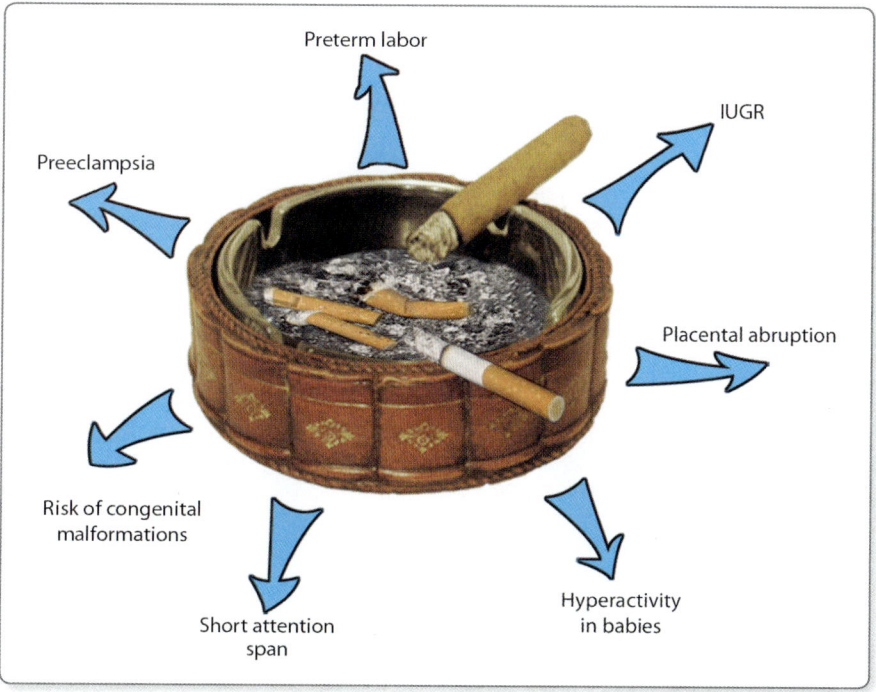

Flow Chart 2.1   Adverse effect of smoking tobacco during pregnancy

Maternal and fetal effects due to smoking tobacco during pregnancy	
Maternal	Fetal
Preeclampsia and abruption placentae	Low birth-weight babies (preterm and intrauterine growth retardation)
Ectopic pregnancy	Risk of congenital anomalies
Miscarriage	Short attention span and hyperactivity
Abnormal placental attachment resulting in placenta previa	Reduced IQ and cognitive performance
Vaginal bleeding	Developmental and behavioral abnormalities in the child
Suppression of lactation	

Adverse effect of smoking tobacco during pregnancy on mother and fetus

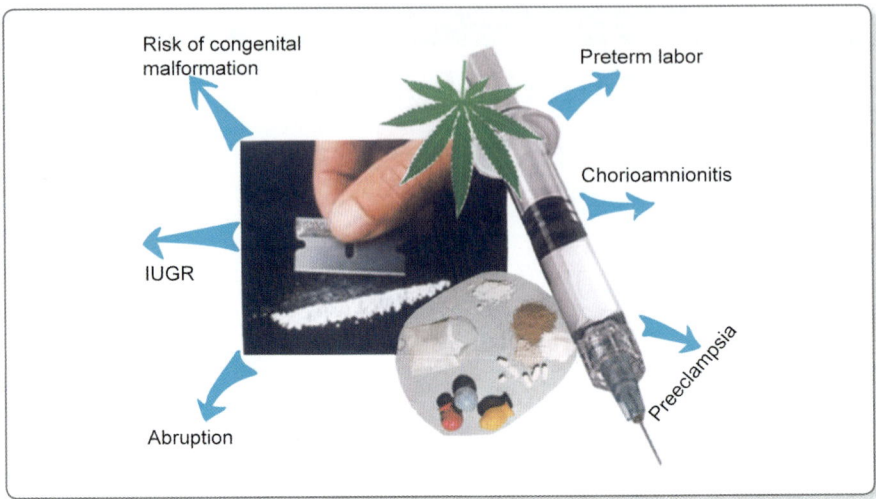

Flow Chart 2.2 Maternal and fetal complications associated with drug abuse during pregnancy

Classifications of various commonly used drugs

Drug category	Examples	Main effect produced
Central nervous system stimulants	Amphetamines, cocaine, dextroamphetamine, methamphetamine and methylphenidate (Ritalin®)	These drugs have a stimulating effect over the central nervous system
Central nervous system depressants	Barbiturates (amobarbital, pentobarbital, secobarbital), benzodiazepine (Valium®, Ativan®, Xanax®), chloral hydrate, alcohol, gamma hydroxybutyric acid, etc.	These substances depress the central nervous system resulting in sedation (drowsiness) and reduction of anxiety
Hallucinogens	D-lysergic acid diethyl amide, psilocybin, psilocin (magic mushrooms) and ecstasy	These drugs have hallucinogenic properties and result in hallucinations
Opiates and narcotics	Heroin, opium, codeine, meperidine (Demerol®), hydromorphone (Dilaudid®), oxycodone, etc.	These drugs are powerful painkillers, which have sedative action and also produce a feeling of well-being and elation
Tetrahydrocannabinol	Cannabis, marijuana and hashish	They mainly produce relaxation. However they can also produce some anxiety and paranoid behavior

Classification of various commonly used drugs depending on their chemical composition and action produced

Source: US National Institute on Drug Abuse (NIDA) (2007). Commonly abused drugs. National Institute on Drug Abuse. [Online] Available from http://www.nida.nih.gov/DrugPages/DrugsofAbuse.html [Accessed Dec, 2012]

3. Common Pregnancy-Related Problems

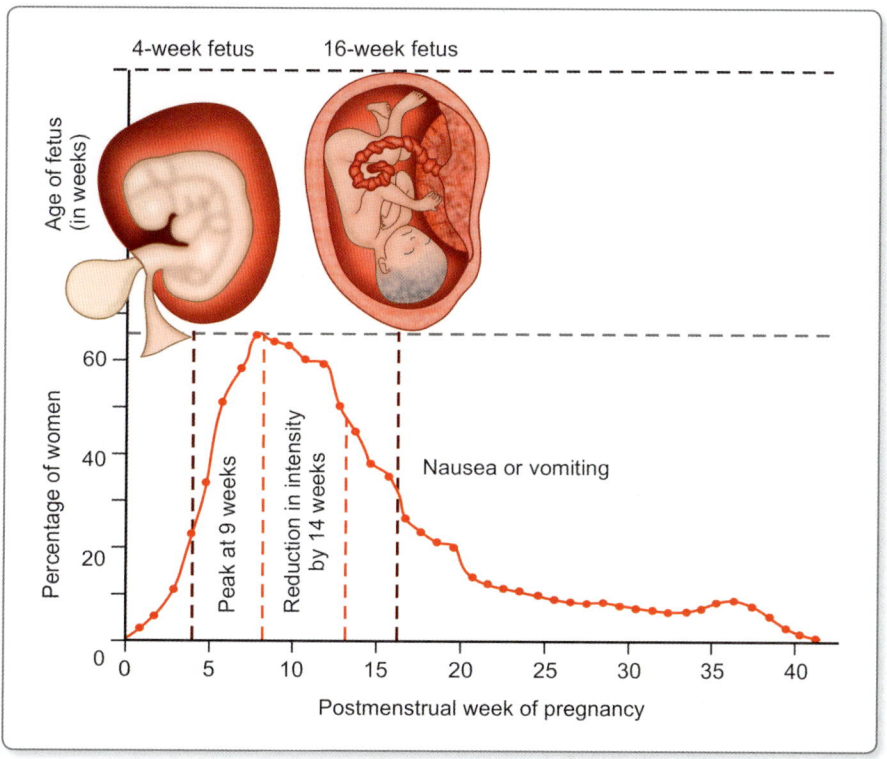

Pattern of morning sickness during pregnancy

Morning sickness during pregnancy
Morning sickness refers to the common problem of nausea and vomiting which affects majority of pregnant women. It is generally a mild, self-limited condition, commonly encountered between 4th and 7th week of pregnancy, peaking at approximately 9th week of pregnancy and diminishing greatly in intensity by 14–16 weeks of pregnancy. It usually diminishes in intensity by the time the woman approaches the 2nd trimester. Severe form of morning sickness is called hyperemesis and requires medical attention.

Definition of morning sickness during pregnancy

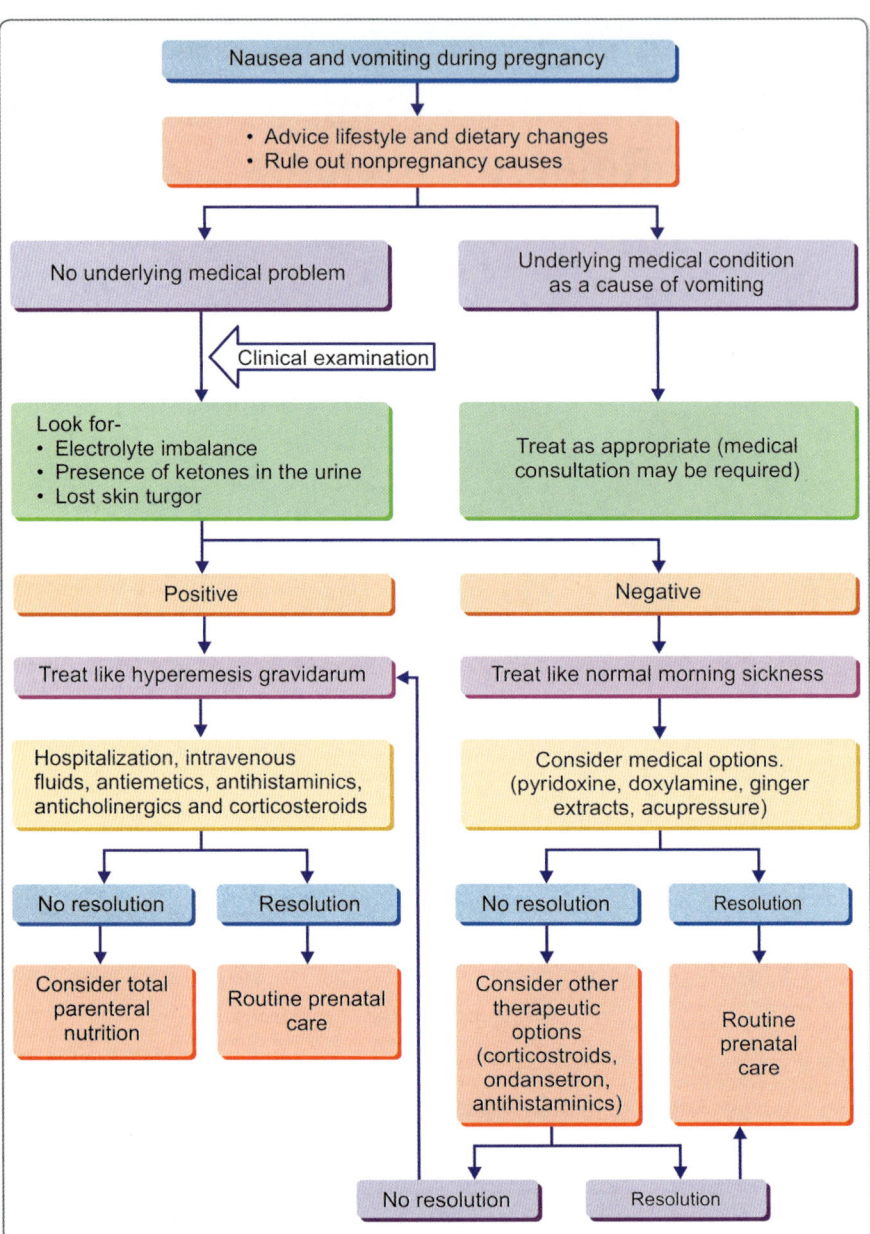

Flow Chart 3.1 Evaluation and management of women with nausea and vomiting during pregnancy

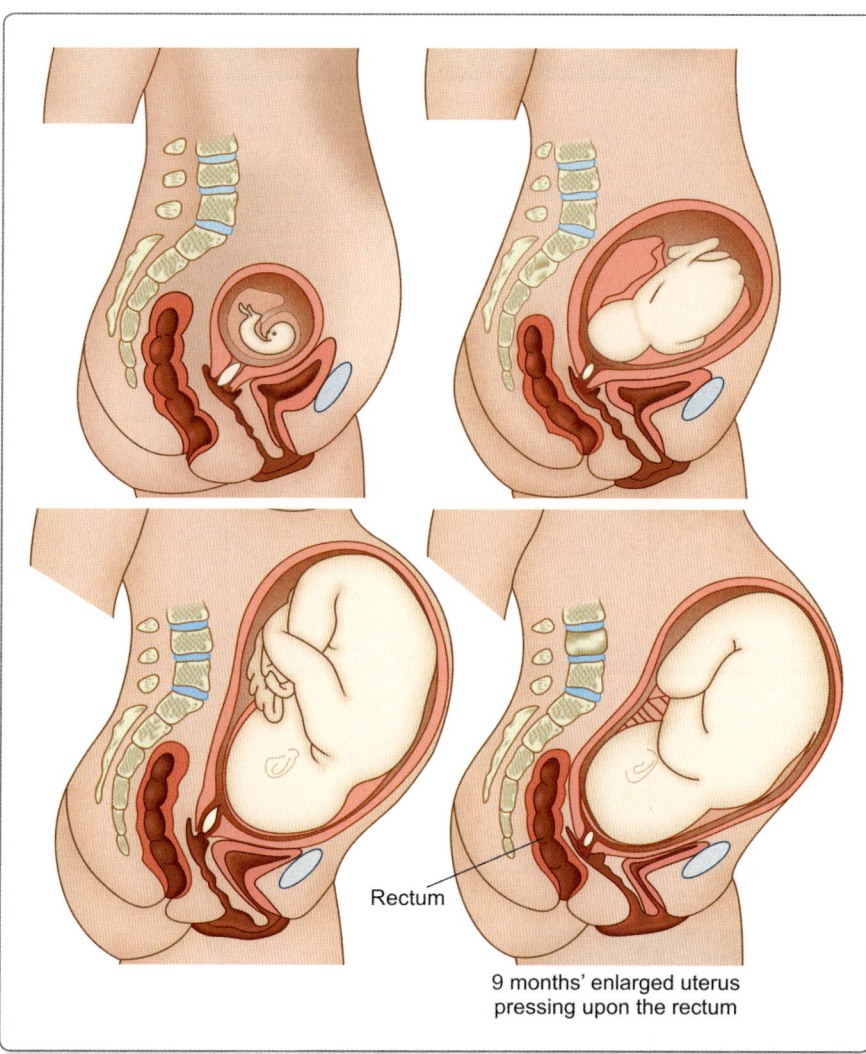

Development of constipation during pregnancy

Causes of constipation in pregnancy
- Increase in the levels of circulating progesterone, a smooth muscle relaxant, especially in the mid and late pregnancy
- Reduced physical activity
- In the later stages of pregnancy the enlarged uterus may also press upon rectum resulting in constipation (as shown in the above figure)

Causes for occurrence of constipation during pregnancy

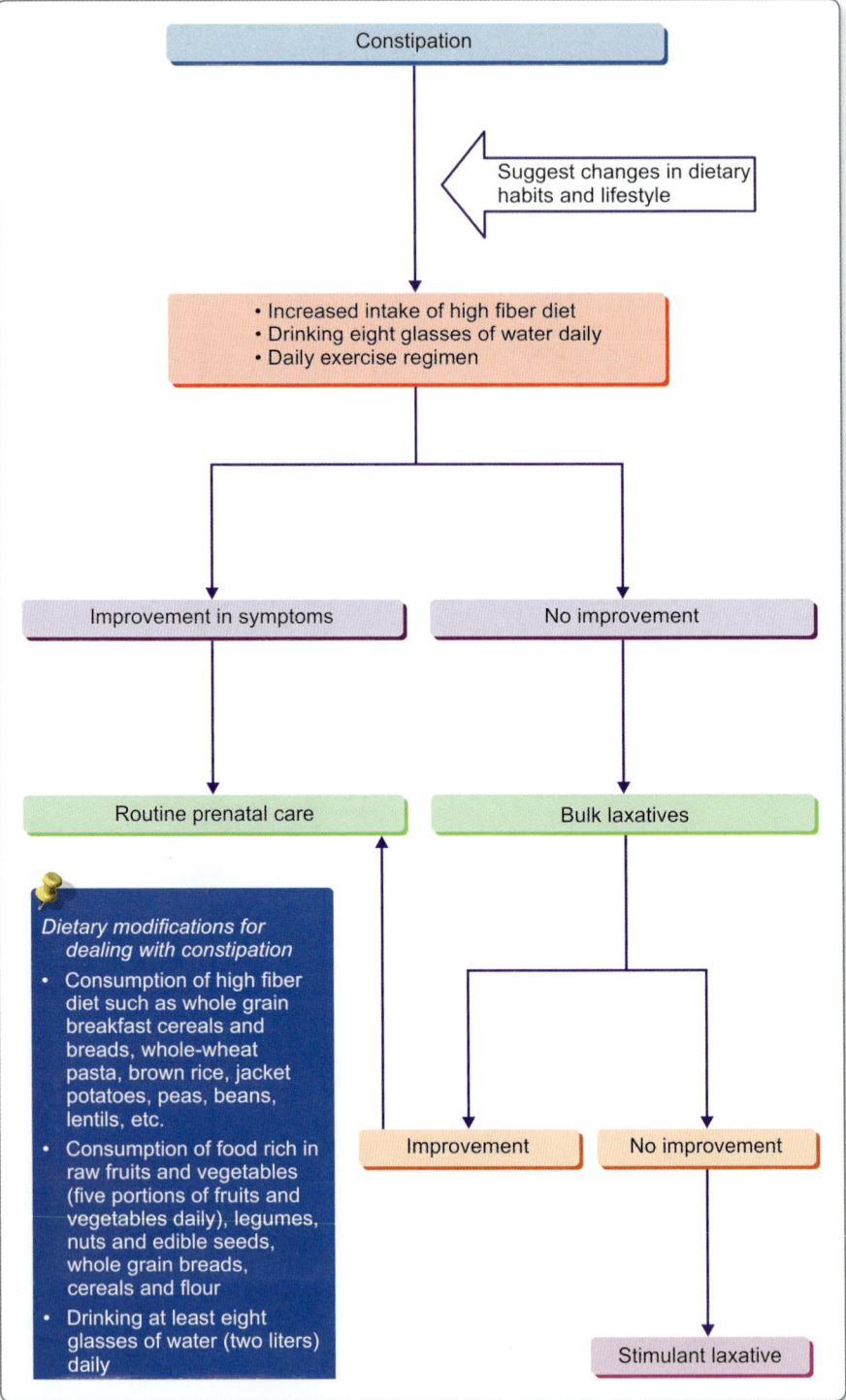

Flow Chart 3.2 Management of constipation during the antenatal period

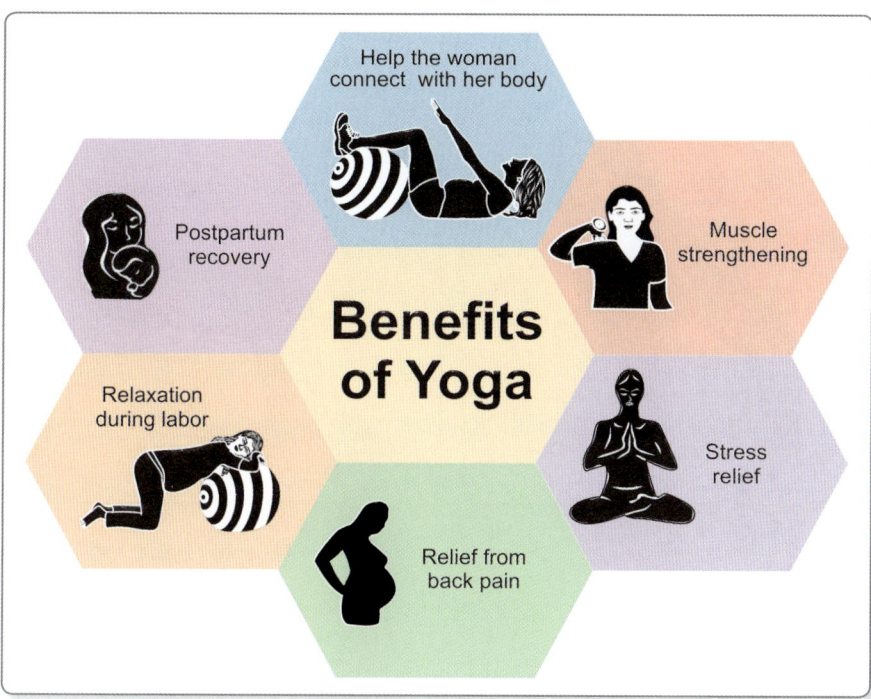

Flow Chart 3.3 Benefits of exercise during pregnancy

Different types of yoga exercises which can be done during pregnancy		
First trimester	Second trimester	Third trimester
• Shavasana • Tadasana • Baddha konasana • Supta baddha konasana • Setubandasana • Pranayamas: anulom vilom breathing and ujjayi breathing	• Tadasana • Trilokasana • Veerasana • Katichakrasana • Dhardasana • Pranayamas: anulom vilom breathing and ujjayi breathing	• Tadasana • Baddha konasana • Setubandhasana • Veerasana • Dandasana • Dhardasana • Pranayams: anulom vilom breathing and ujjayi breathing

Benefits of exercise during pregnancy

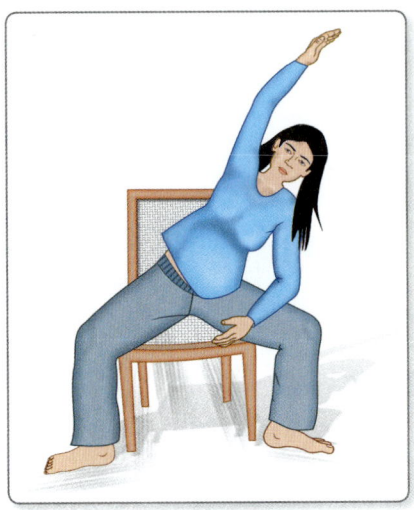
Trilokasana

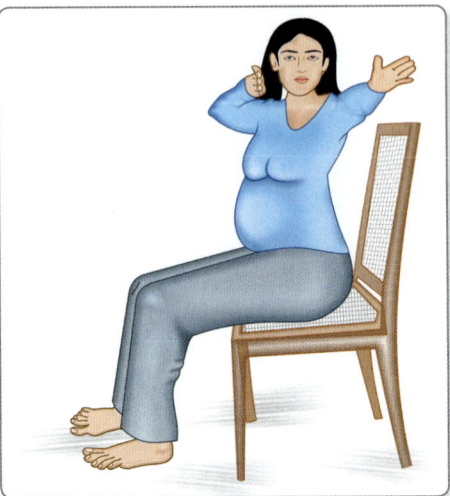
Katichakrasana

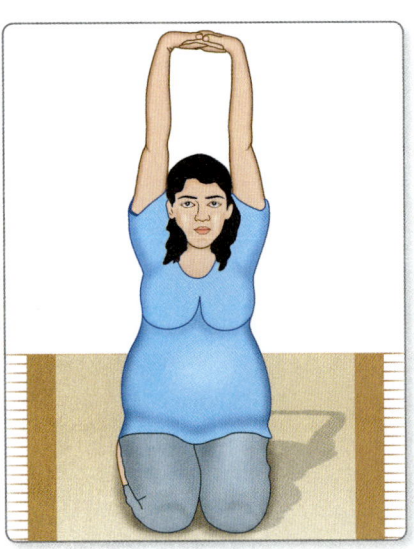
Veerasana

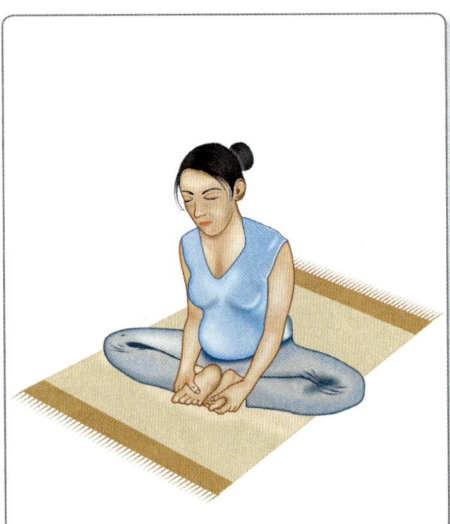
Baddha konasana

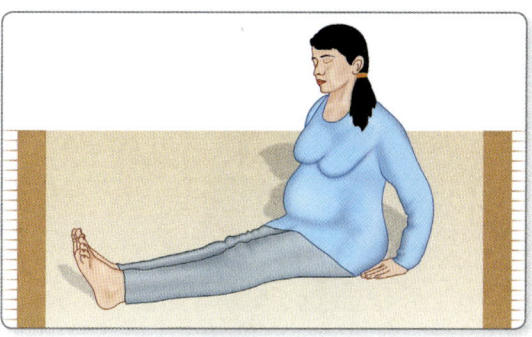
Dandasana

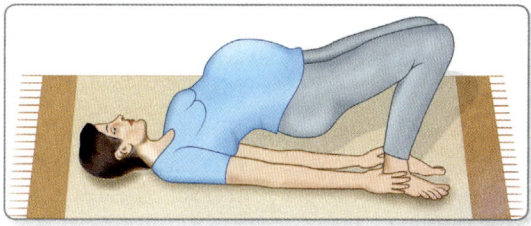
Setubandhasana

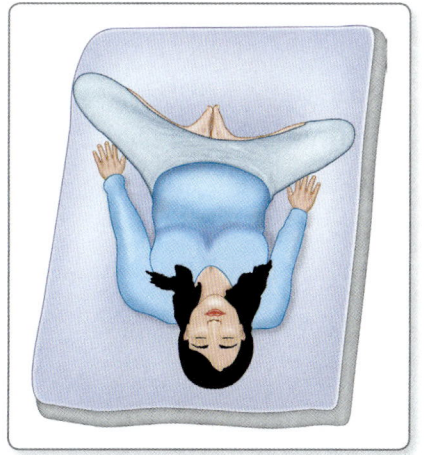
Supta baddha konasana

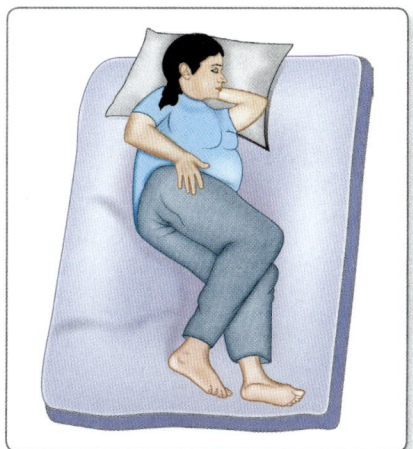
Dhardasana

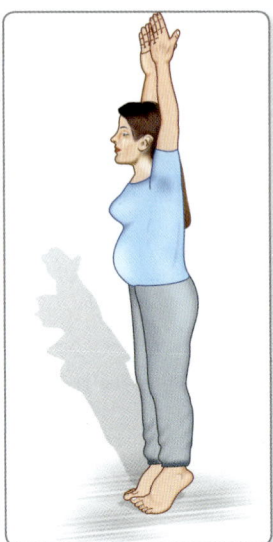

Tadasana

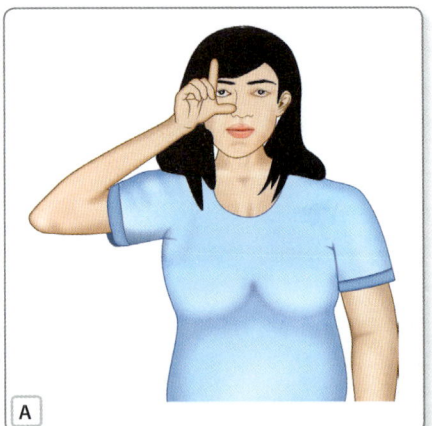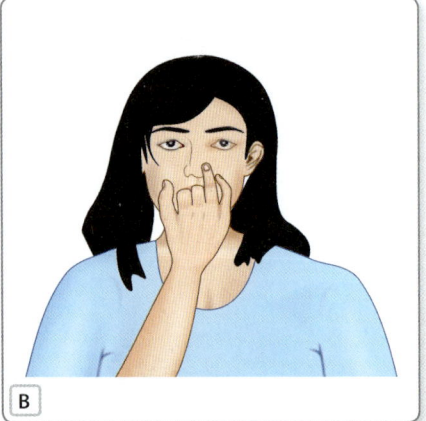

Anulom vilom breathing technique

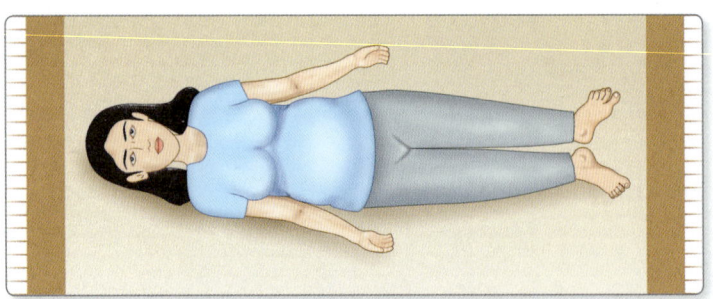

Shavasana

OBSTETRICS

Section 2

Abnormal Presentation

Chapter 4 Breech Presentation
Chapter 5 Transverse Lie

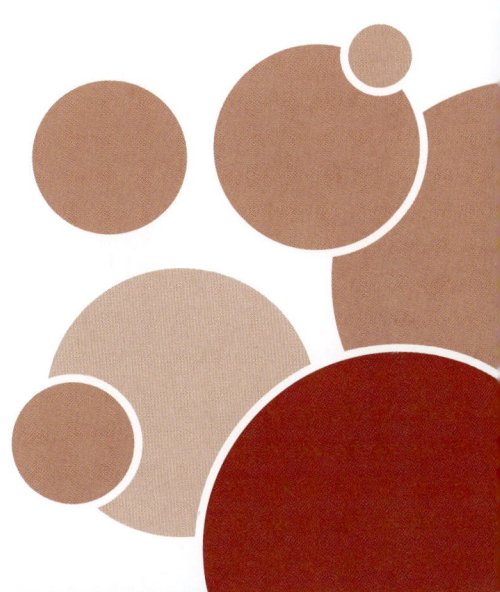

4 Breech Presentation

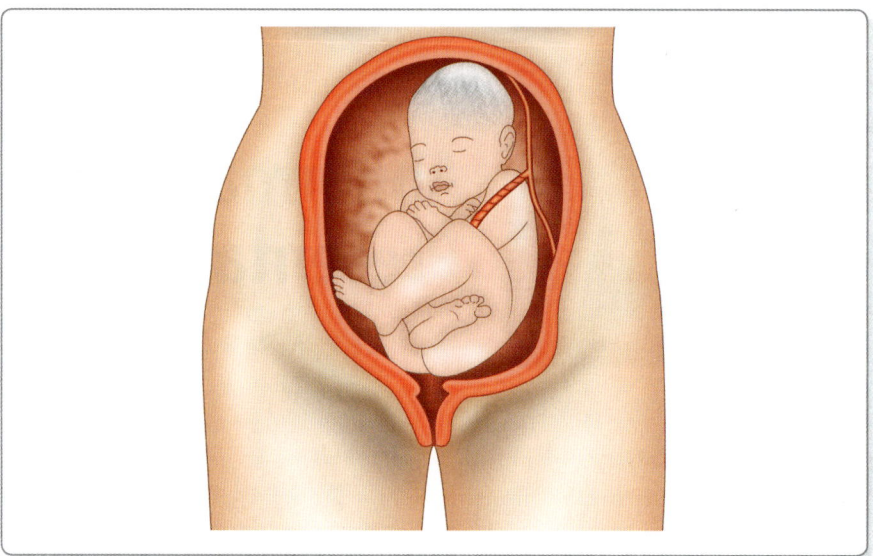

Breech presentation

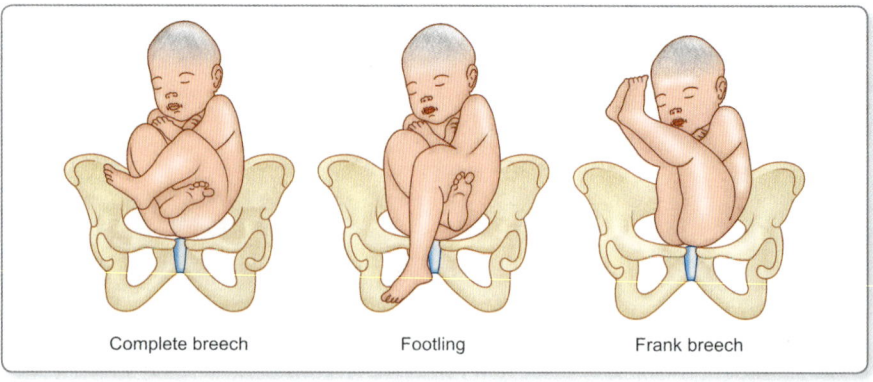

Different types of breech presentation

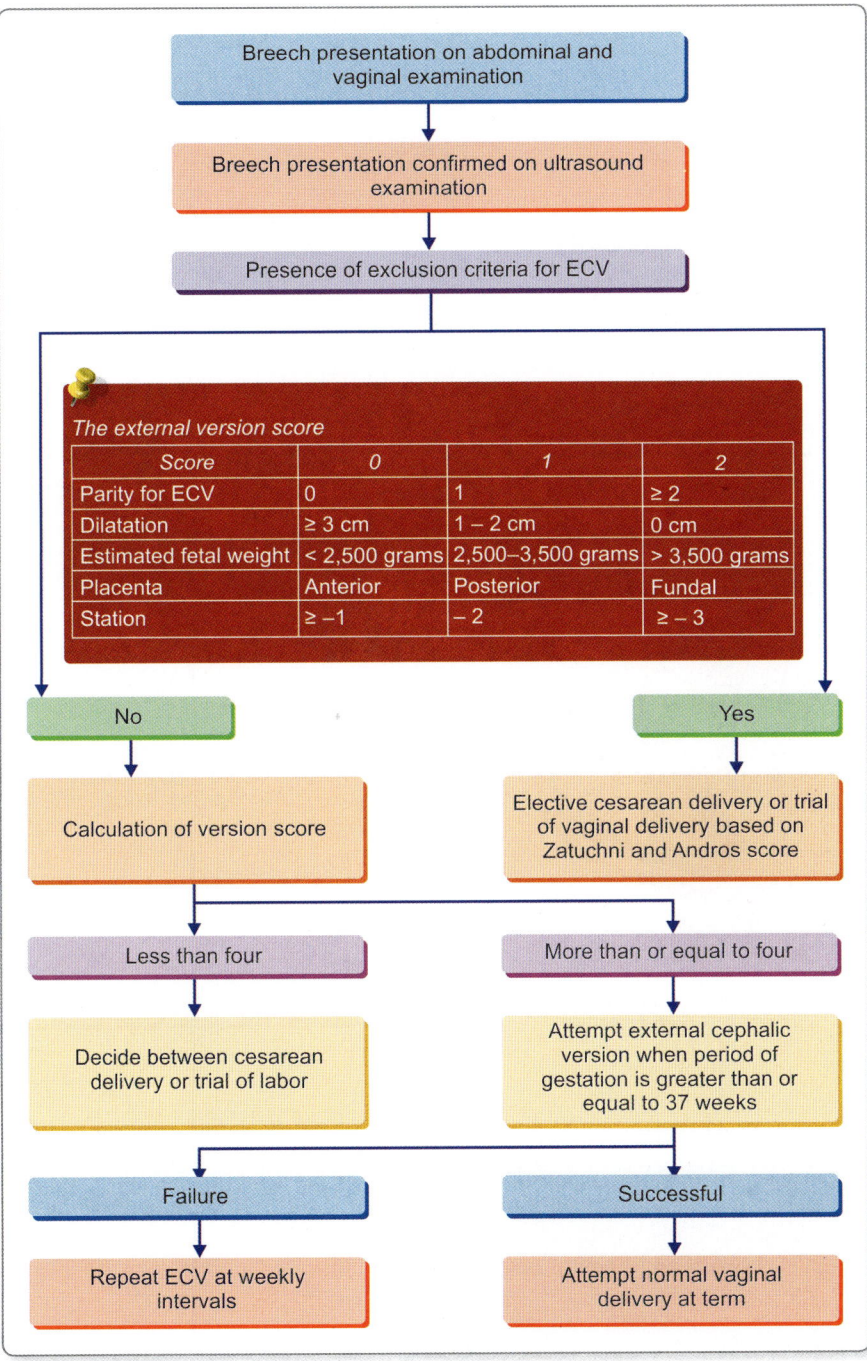

Flow Chart 4.1 Management options for breech presentation

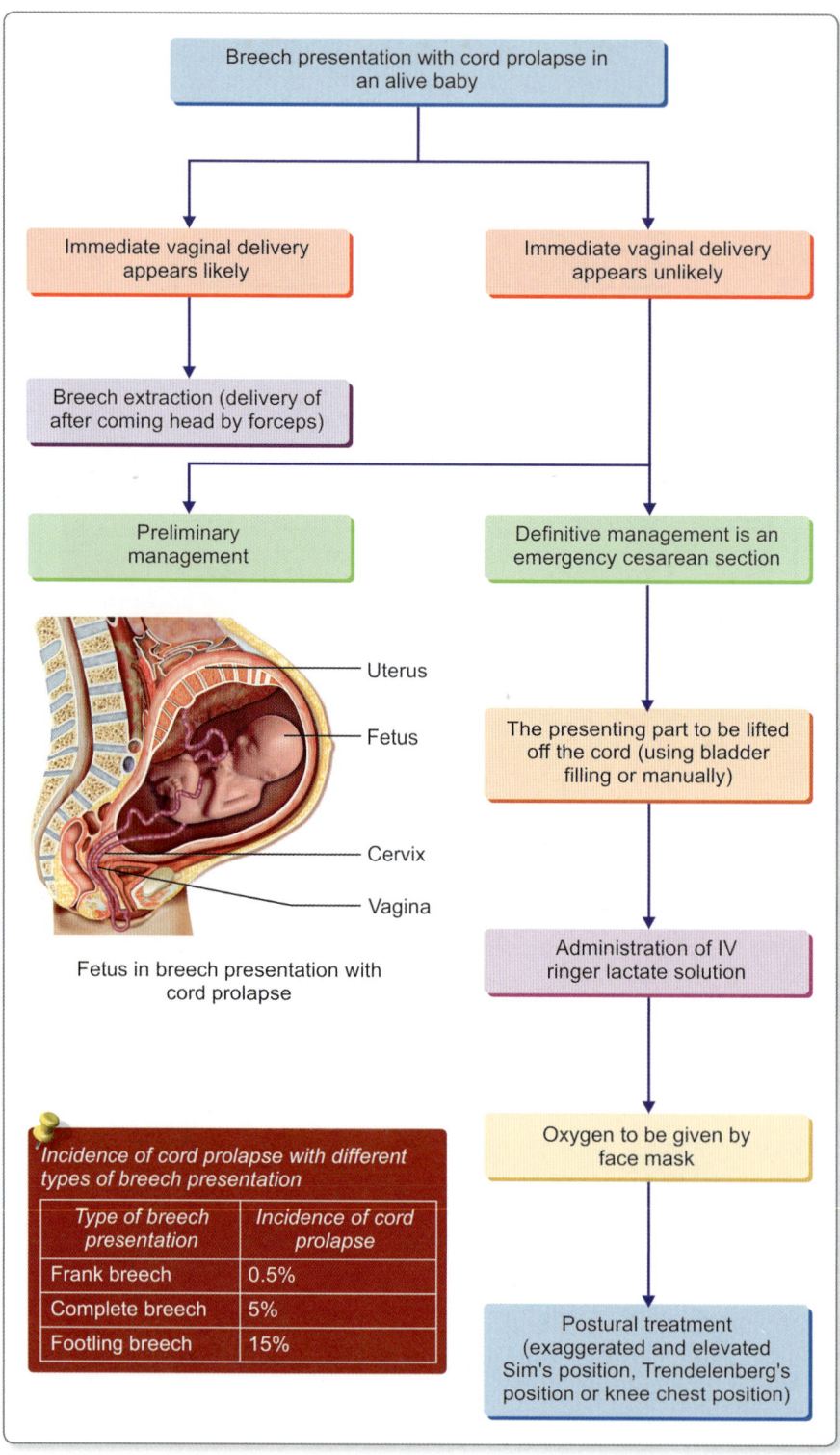

Flow Chart 4.2 Management of cord prolapse

5 Transverse Lie

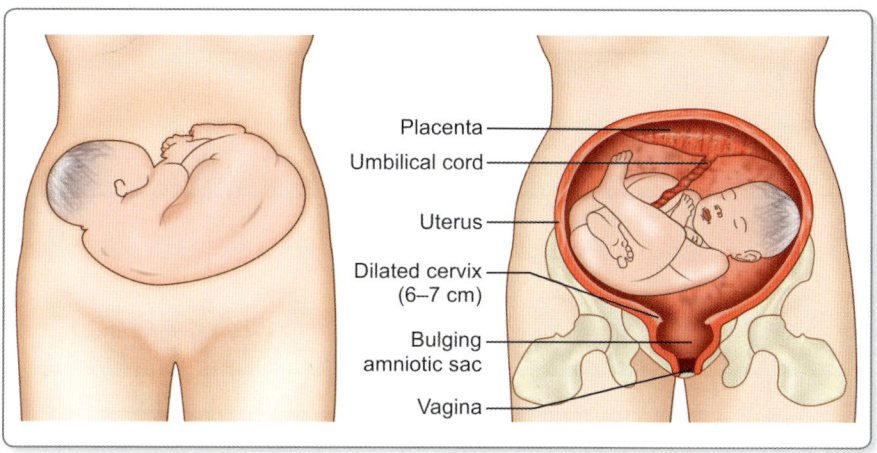

Fetus in transverse lie

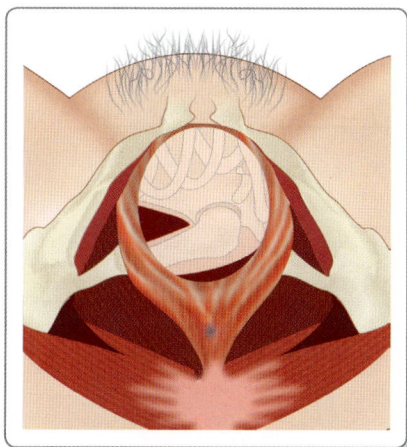

Vaginal touch picture in case of shoulder presentation

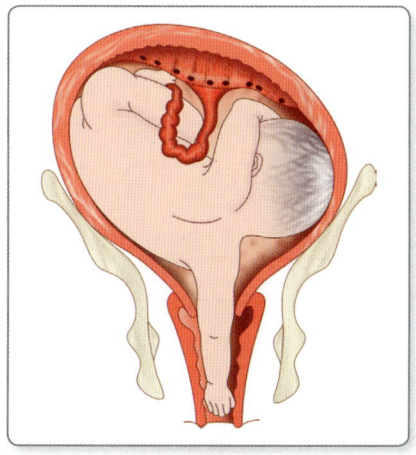

Arm prolapse

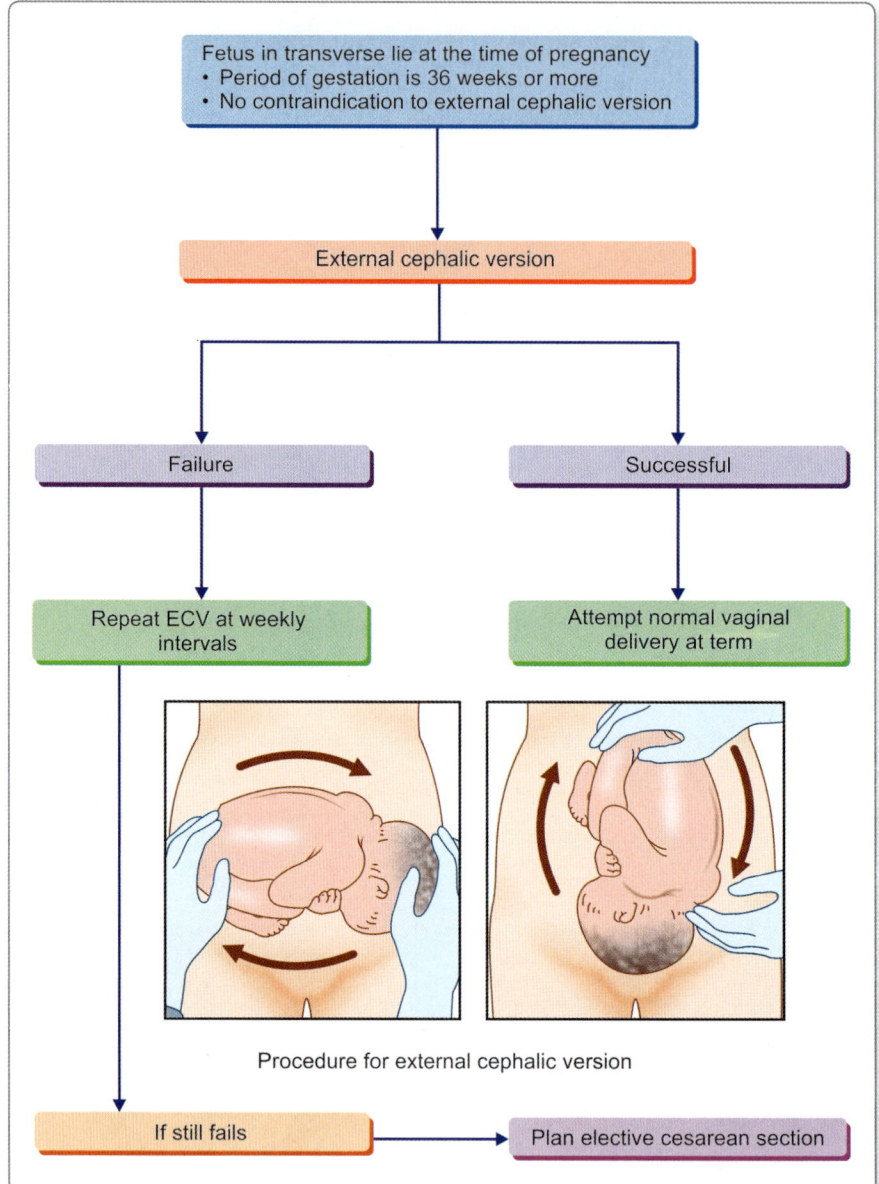

Flow Chart 5.1 Management of a fetus in transverse lie during pregnancy

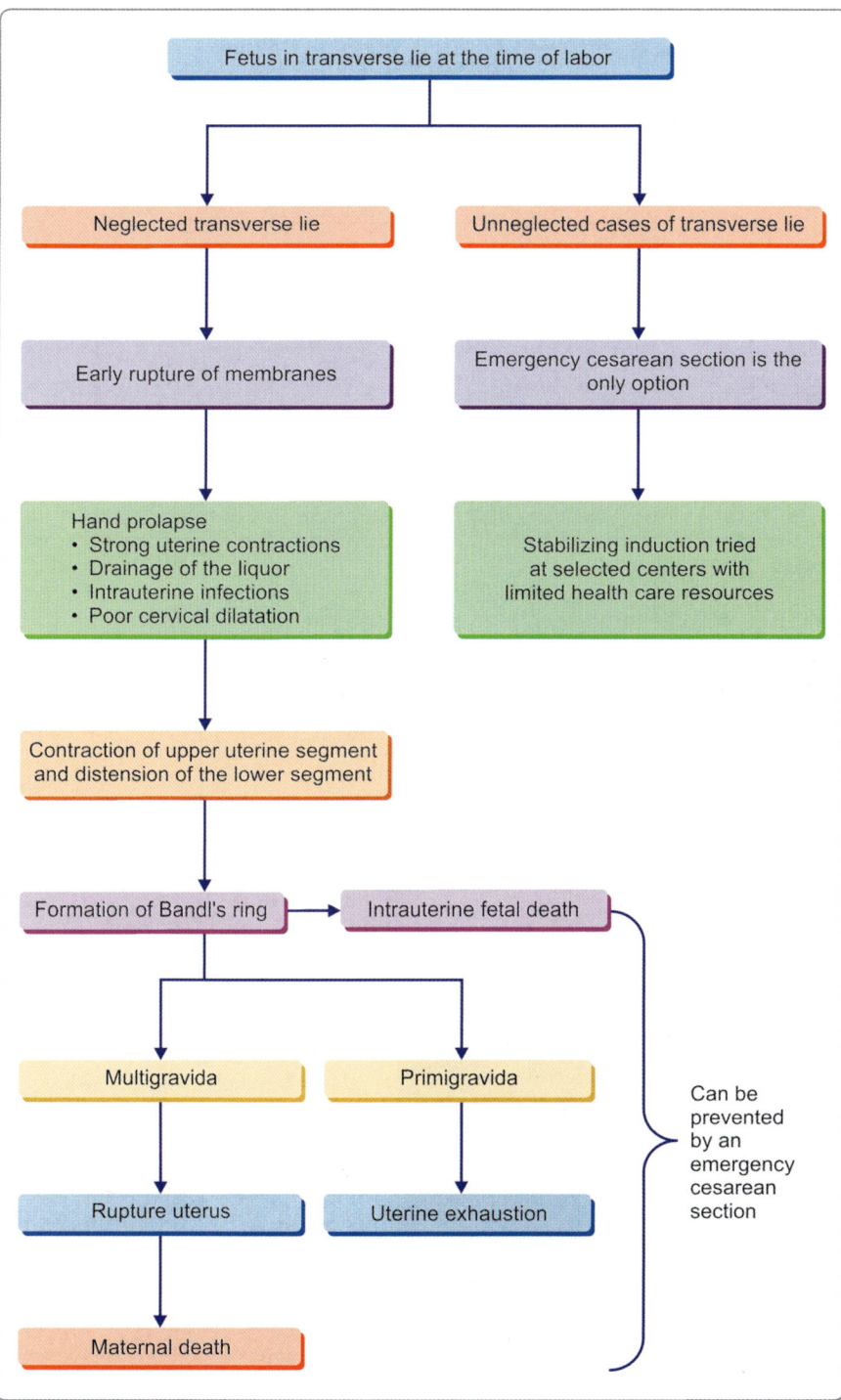

Flow Chart 5.2 Management of a fetus in transverse lie during labor

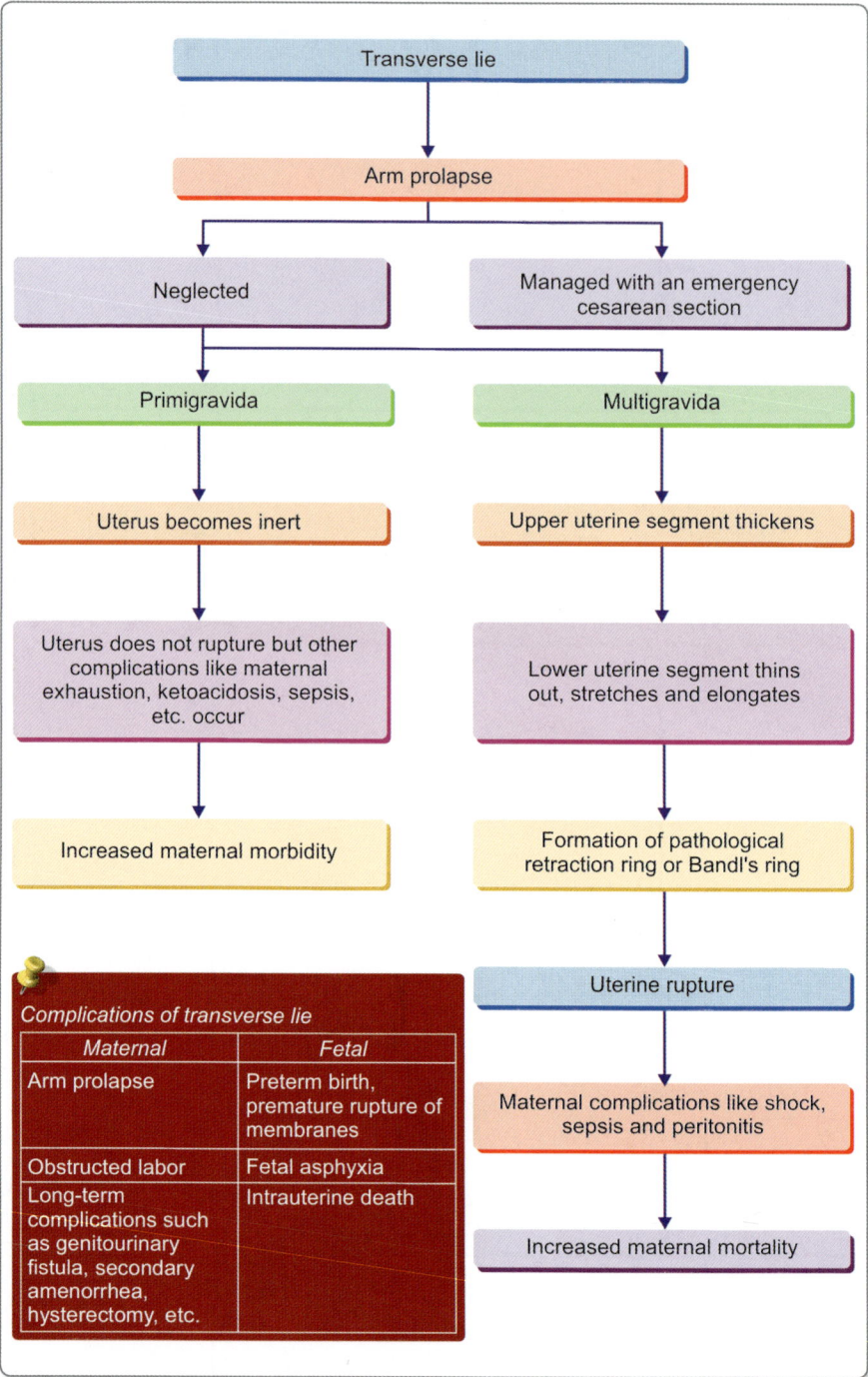

Flow Chart 5.3   Consequences of a neglected arm prolapse

OBSTETRICS

Section 3: Pregnancy-Related Complications

- **Chapter 6** Antepartum Hemorrhage
- **Chapter 7** Twin Pregnancy
- **Chapter 8** Rh-Negative Pregnancy
- **Chapter 9** Hydatidiform Mole
- **Chapter 10** Fetal Growth Restriction
- **Chapter 11** Preterm Pregnancy
- **Chapter 12** Post-Term Pregnancy
- **Chapter 13** Polyhydramnios
- **Chapter 14** Urogenital Fistula Due to Obstructed Labor
- **Chapter 15** Miscarriage
- **Chapter 16** Previous Cesarean Section

6. Antepartum Hemorrhage

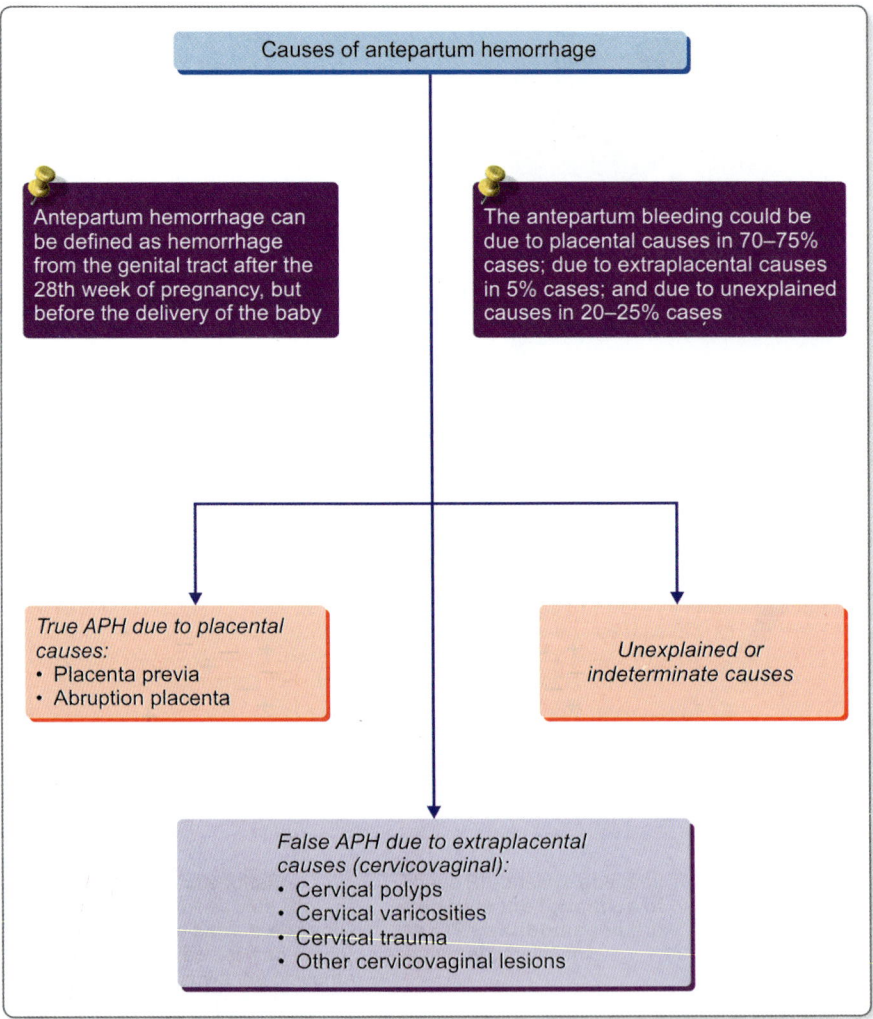

Flow Chart 6.1   Causes of antepartum hemorrhage

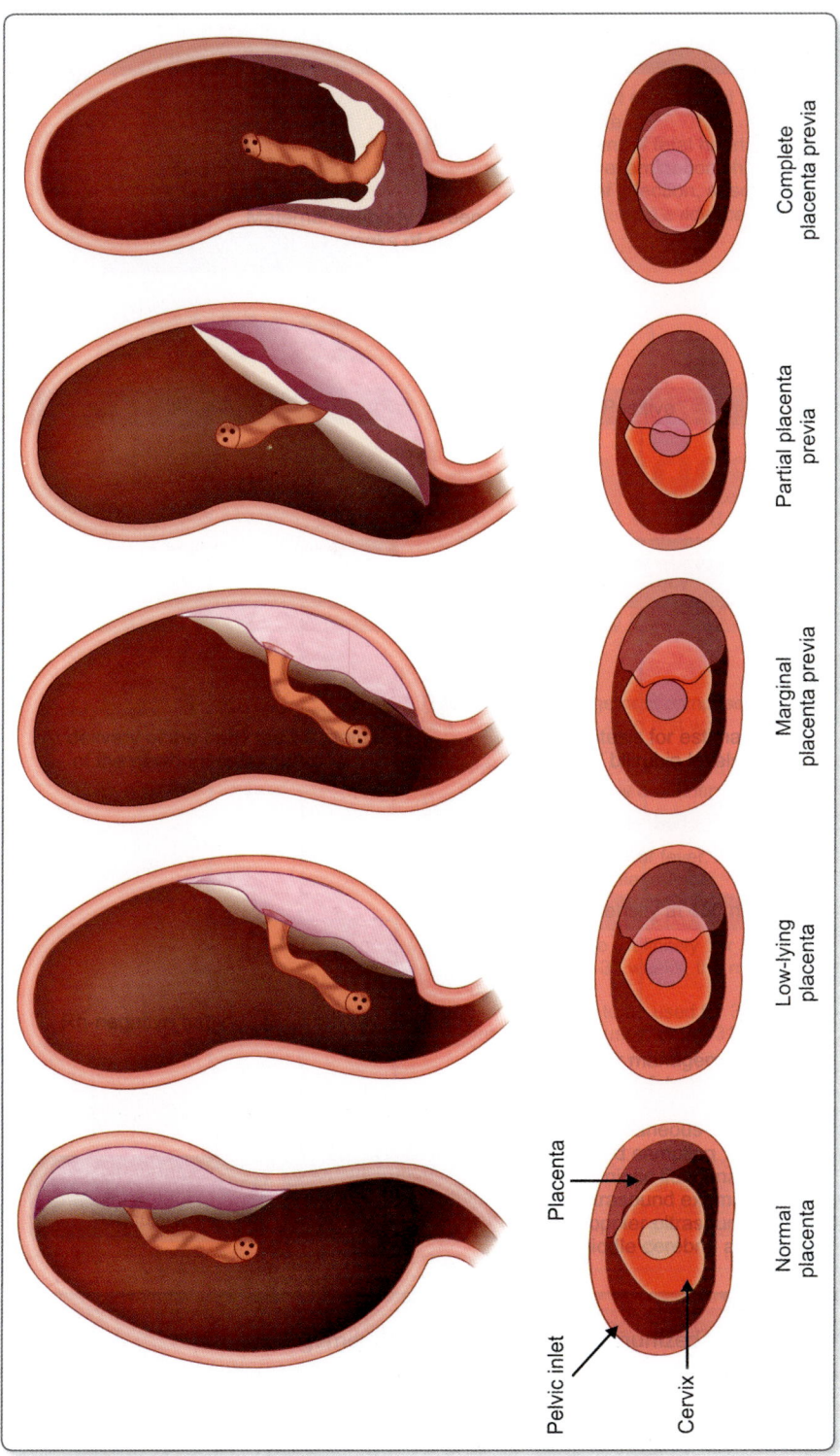

Relationship of various types of placenta previa with cervix

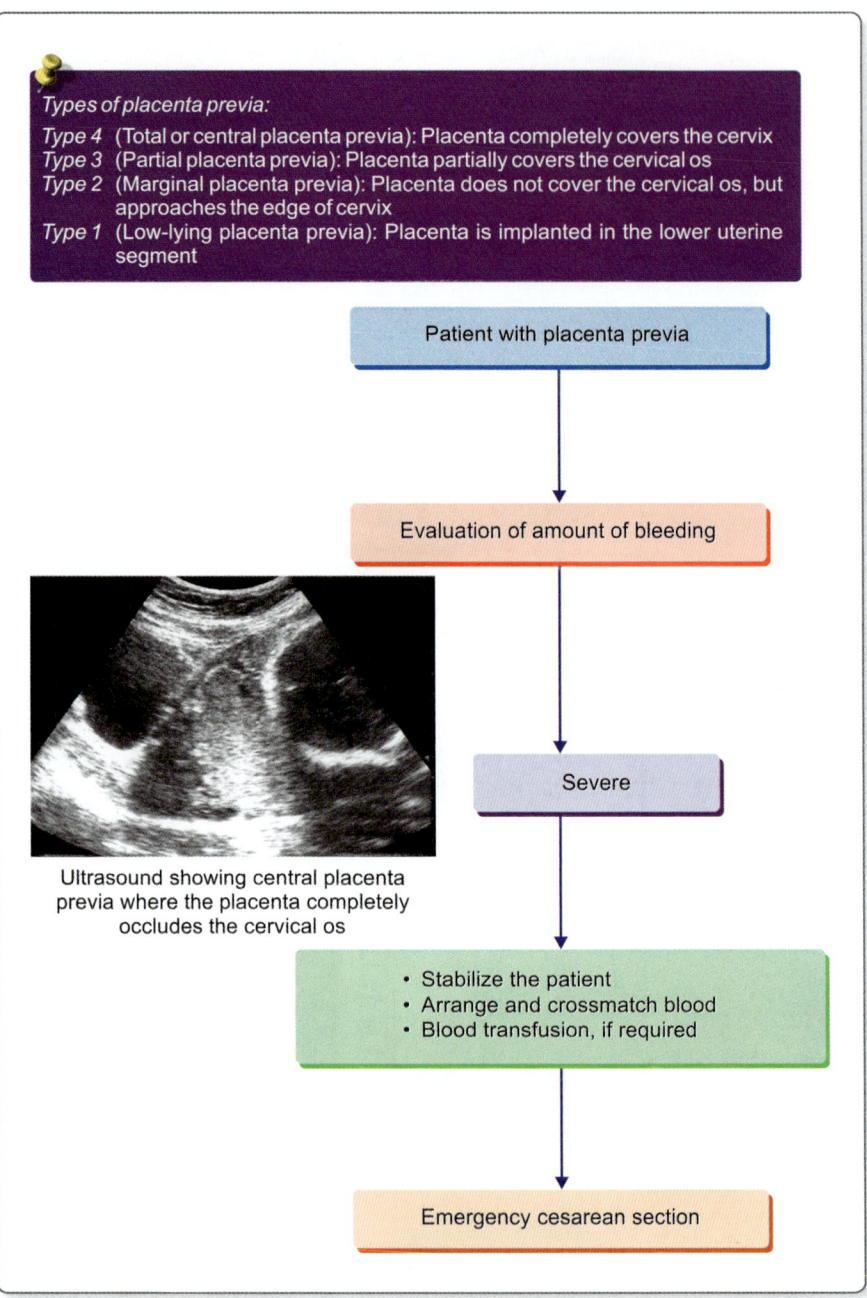

Flow Chart 6.2 Management plan in a patient with severe placenta previa (type 4 and 3)

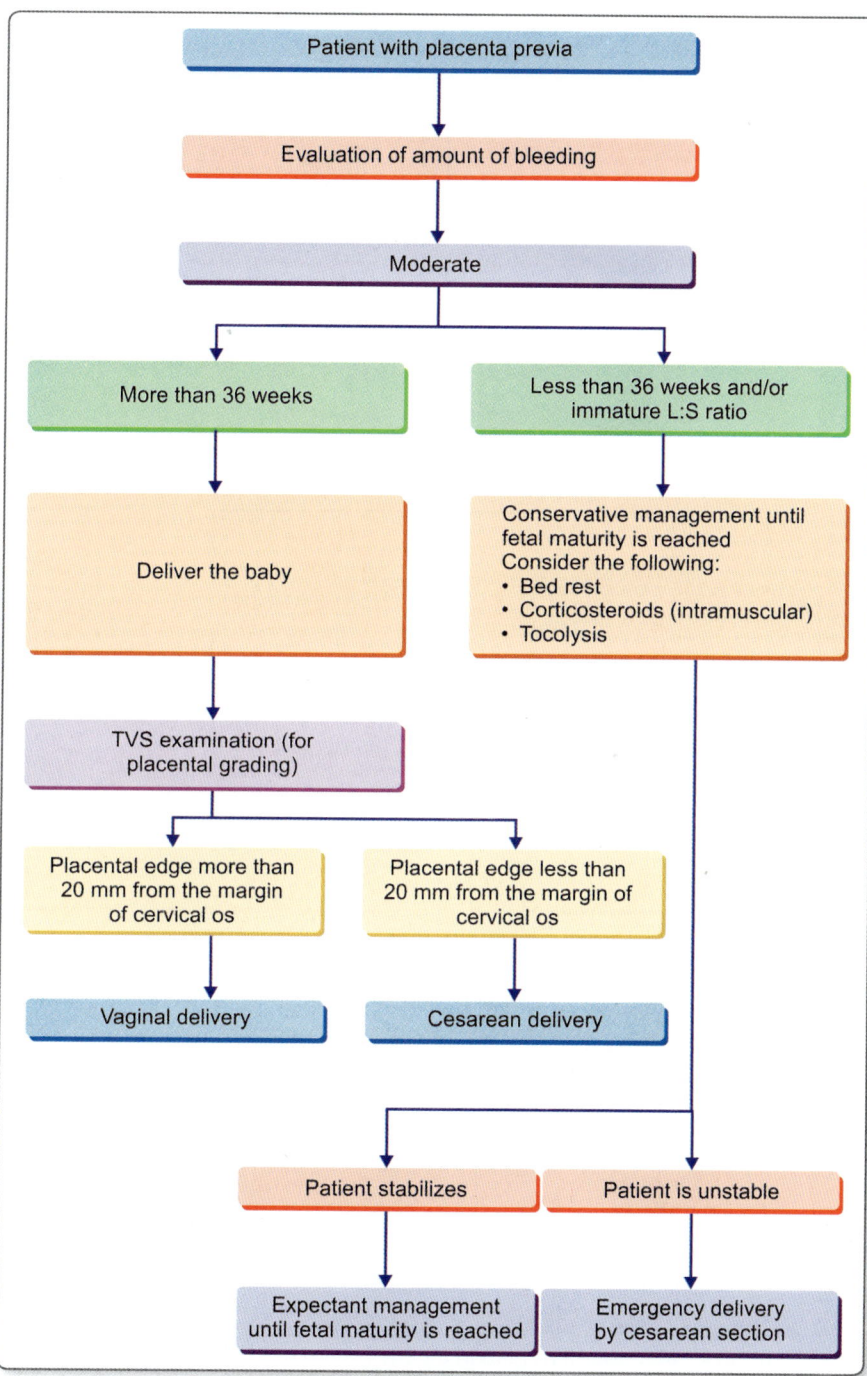

Flow Chart 6.3 Management plan in a patient with moderate placenta previa (type 2)

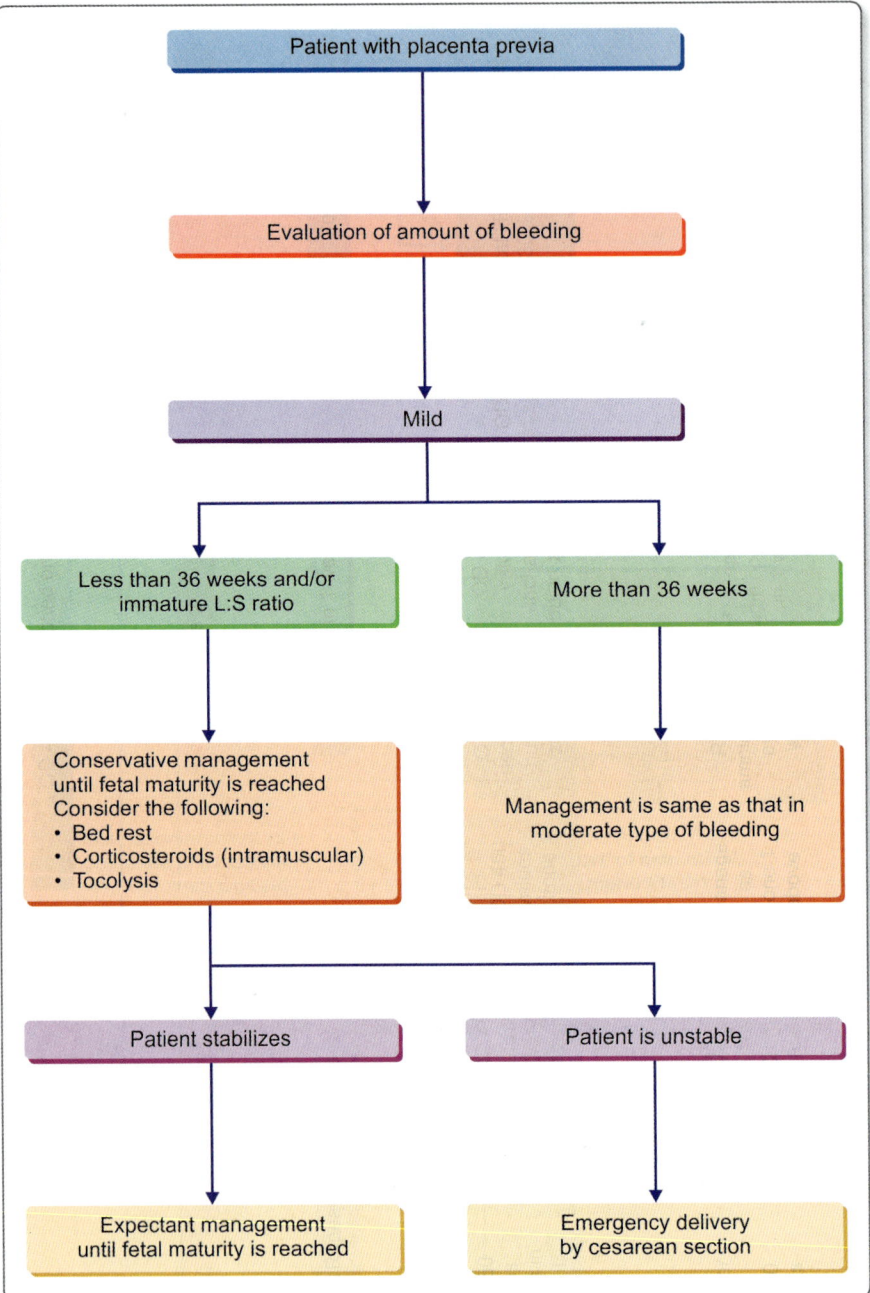

Flow Chart 6.4 Management plan in a patient with mild placenta previa (type 1)

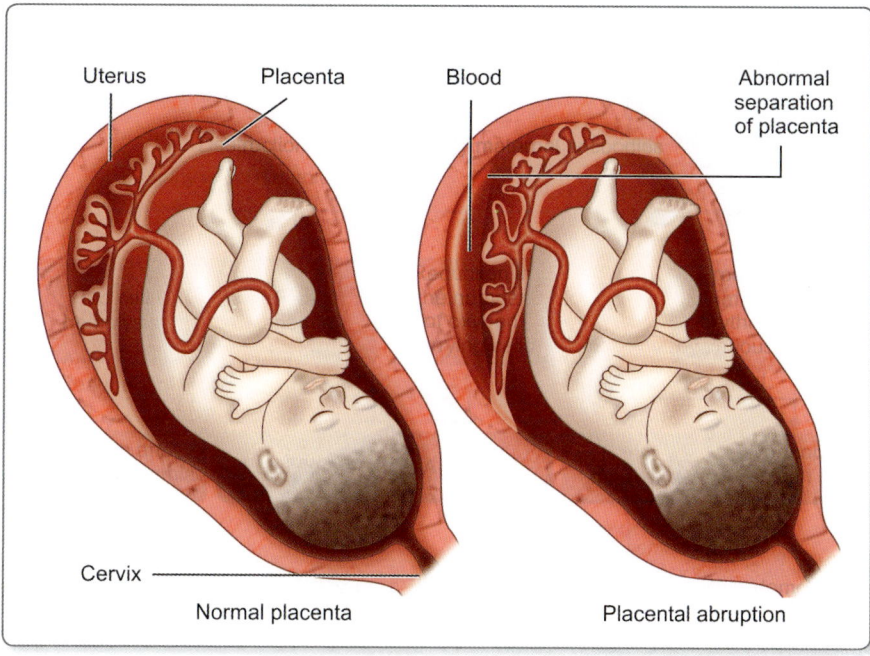

Placental abruption and its comparison with normal placenta

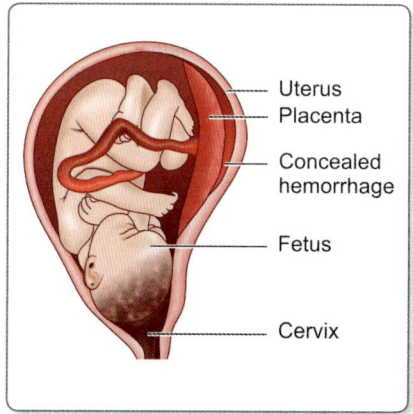

Concealed type of placental abruption

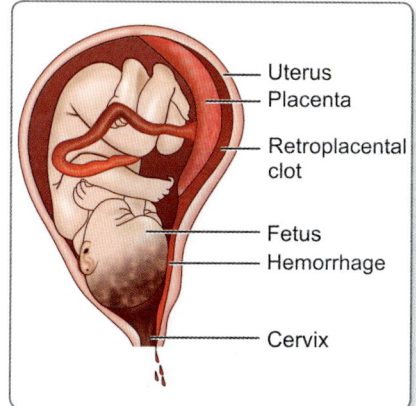

Revealed type of placental abruption

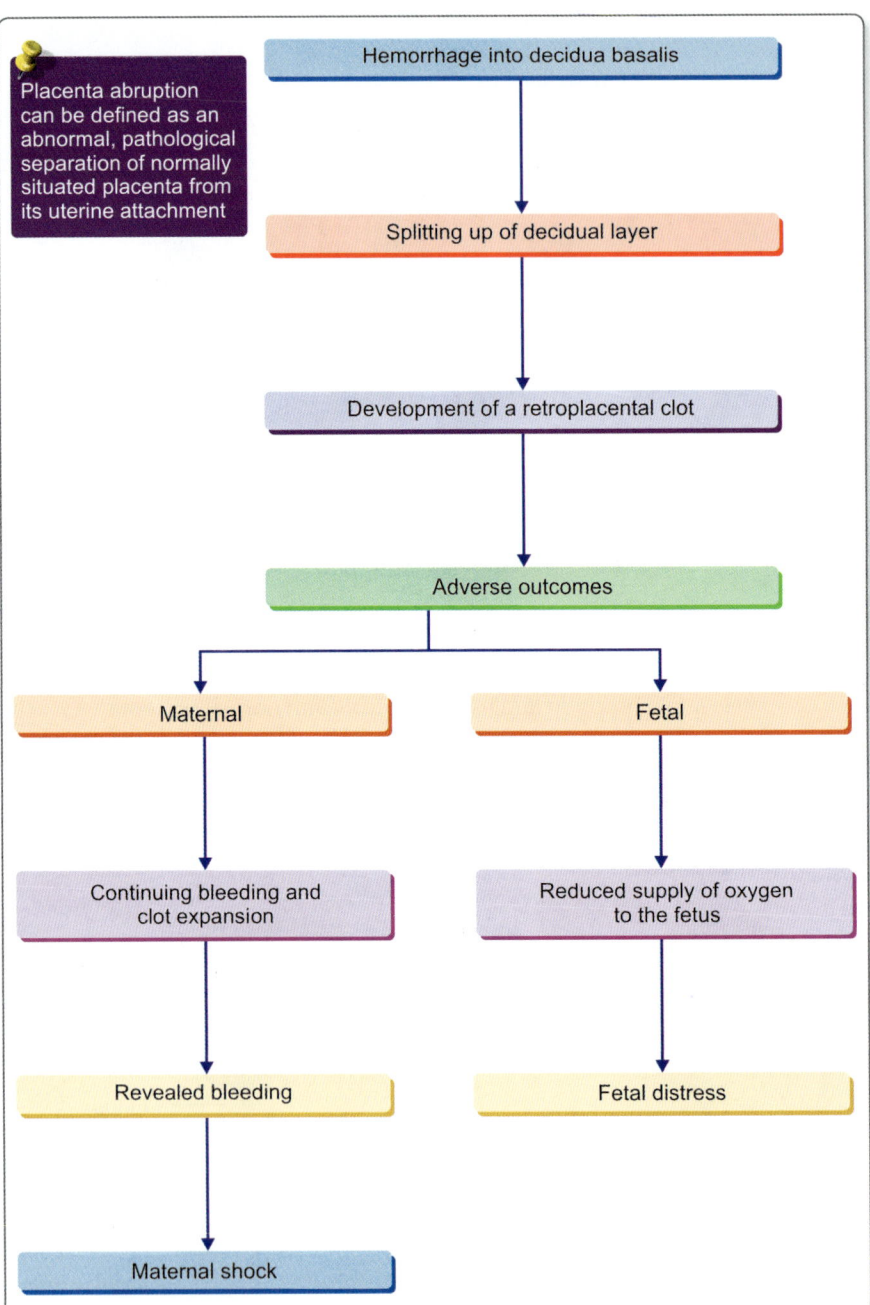

Flow Chart 6.5 Pathophysiology of abruption placenta

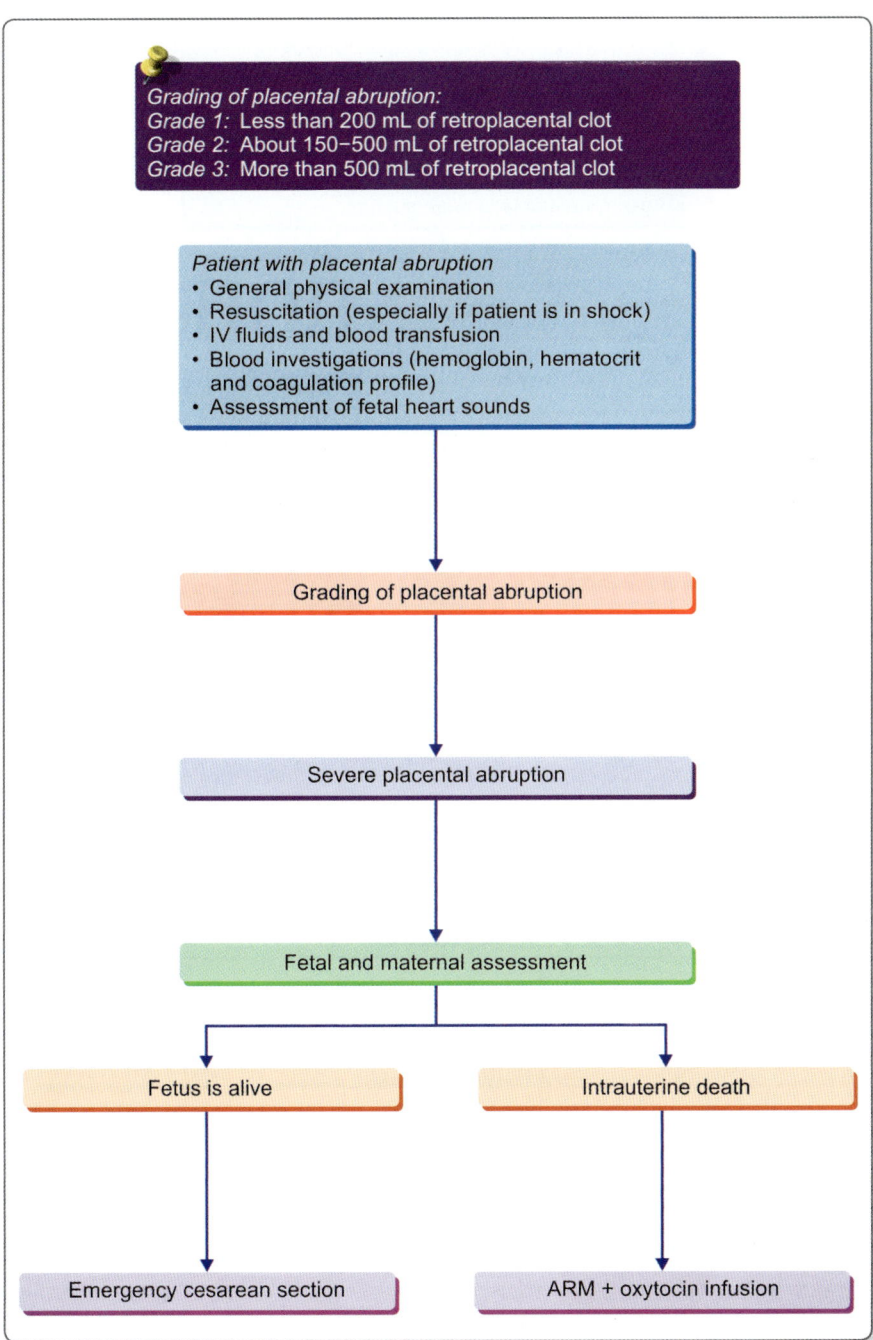

Flow Chart 6.6 Treatment plan of a patient with severe abruption placenta (grade 3)

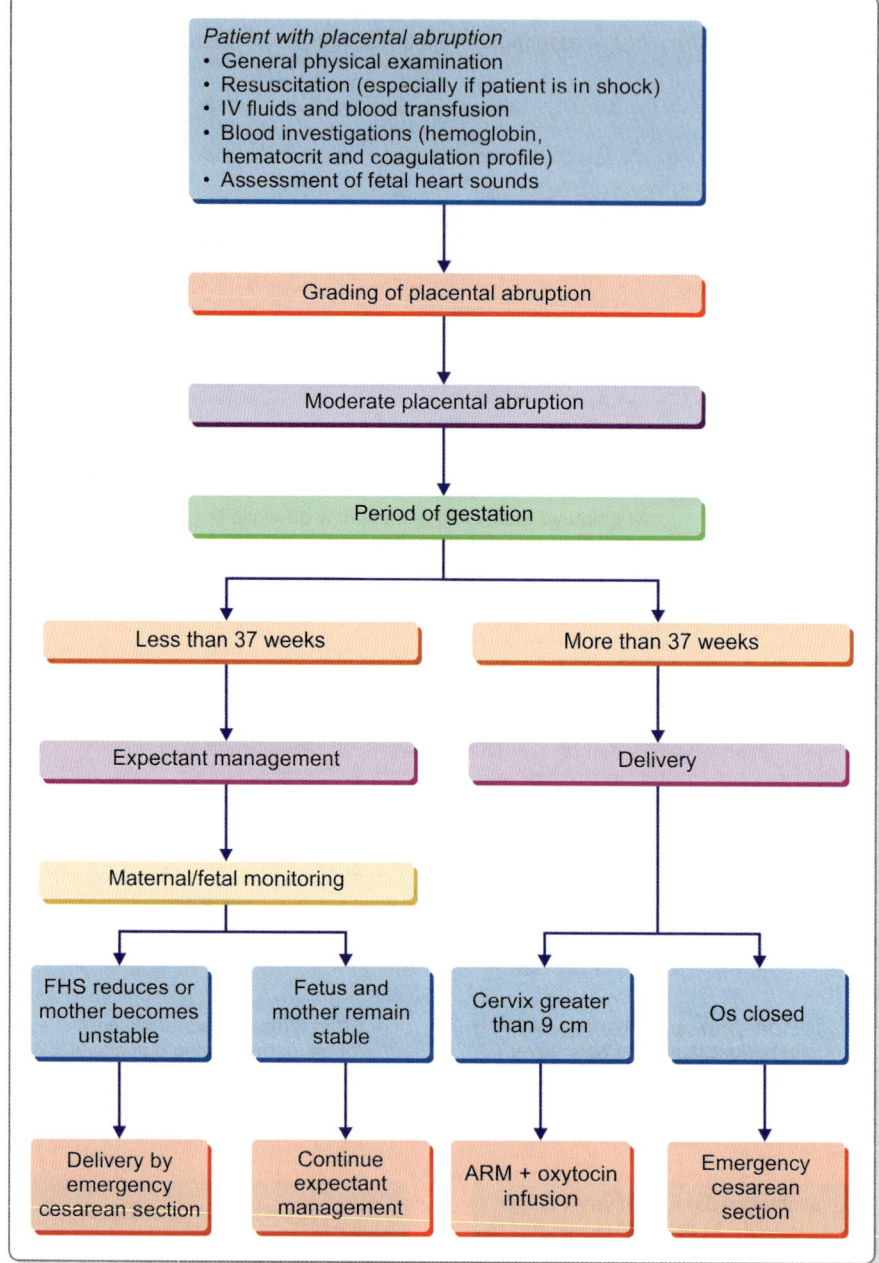

Flow Chart 6.7 Treatment plan of a patient with moderate abruption placenta (grade 2)

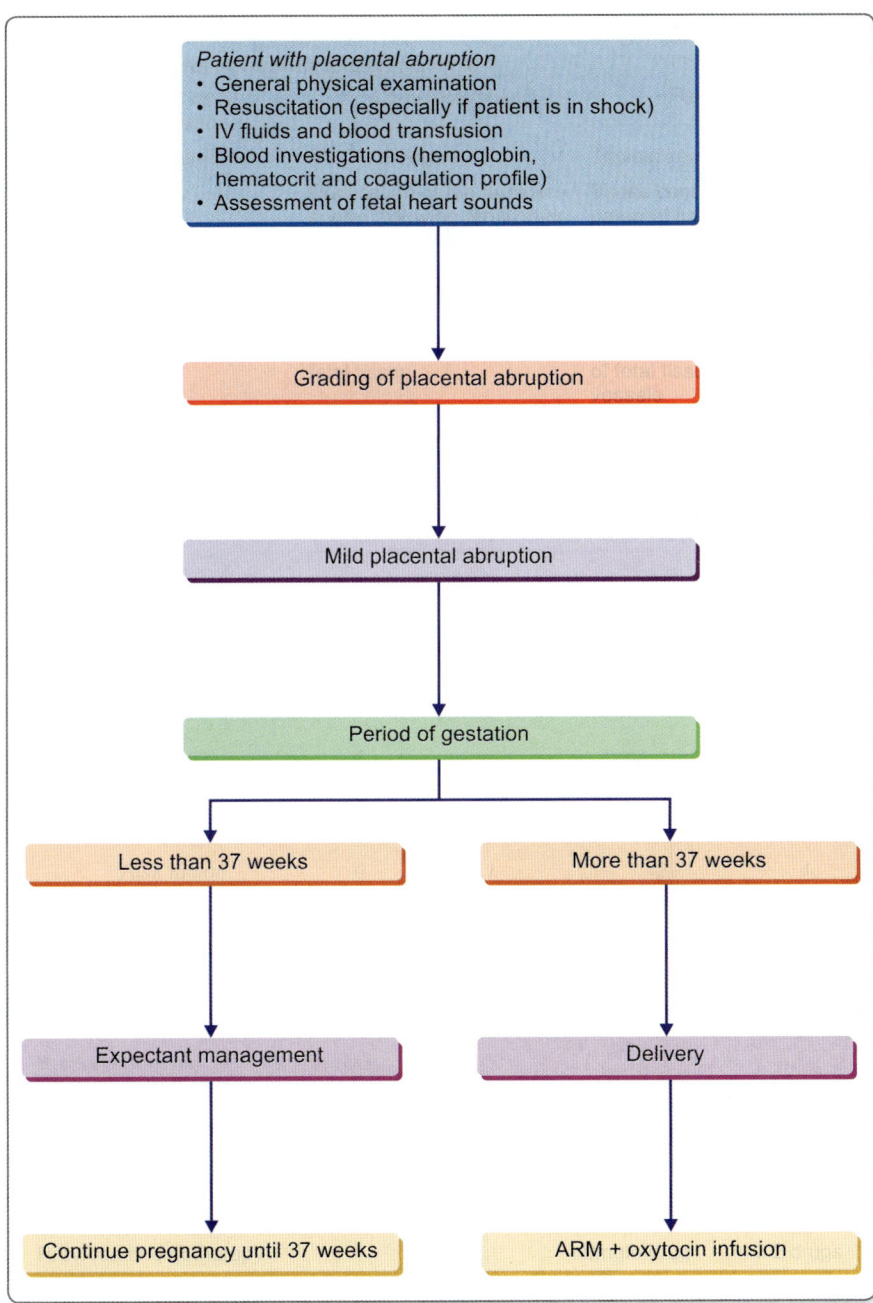

Flow Chart 6.8 Treatment plan of a patient with mild abruption placenta (grade 1)

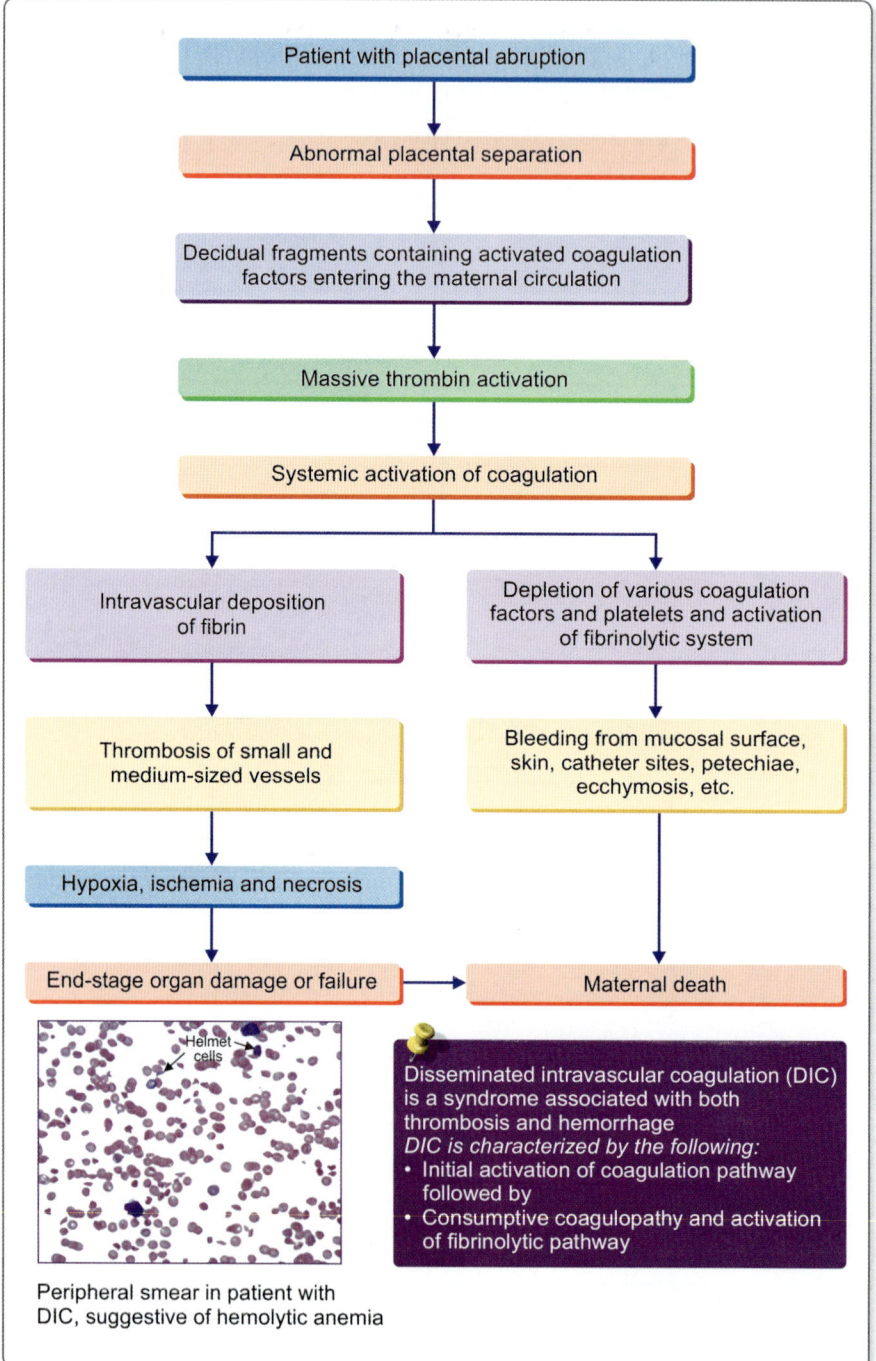

Flow Chart 6.9 Pathogenesis of DIC in cases of abruption placenta

7 Twin Pregnancy

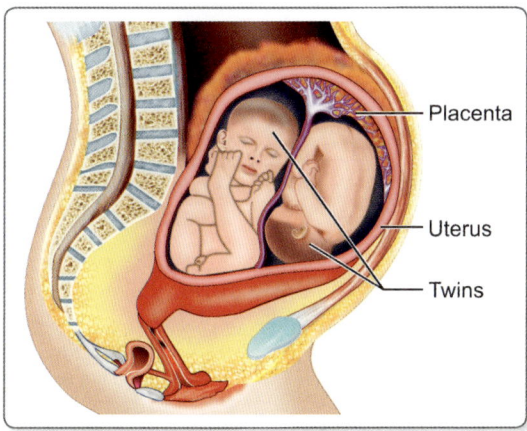

Multifetal gestation: Twin pregnancy

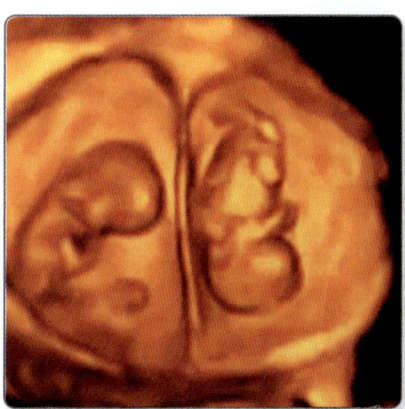

Three-dimensional ultrasound showing diamniotic dichorionic twins at 9 weeks of gestation

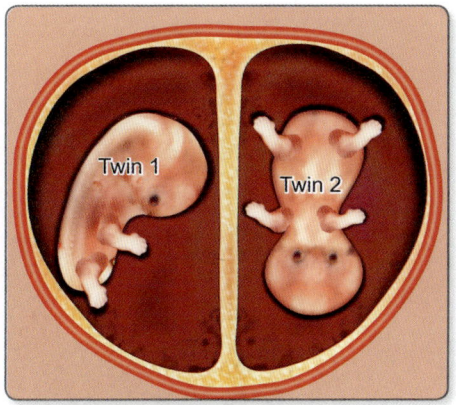

Diagrammatic representation of twins at 9 weeks of gestation

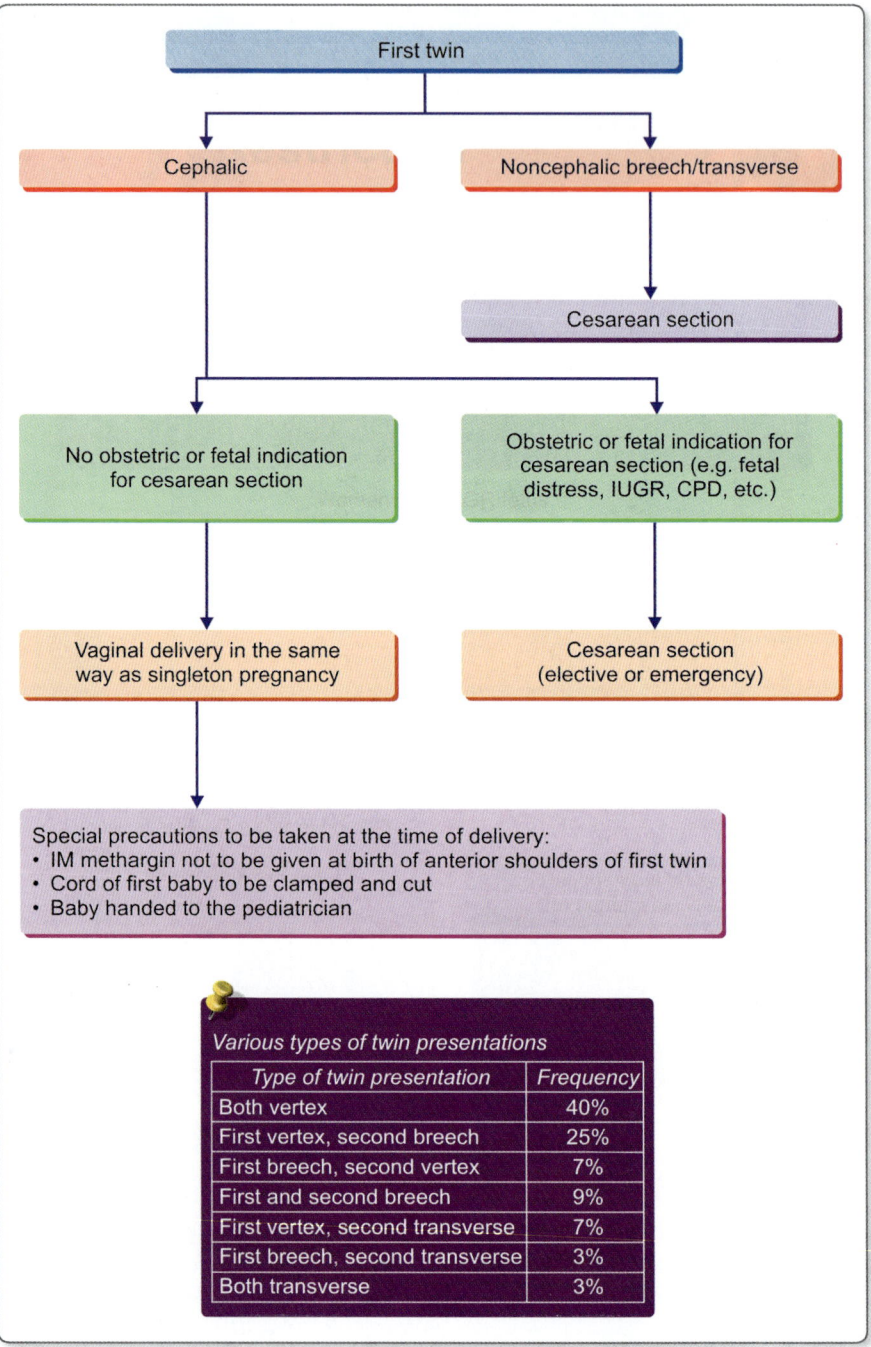

Flow Chart 7.1 Intrapartum management of first twin

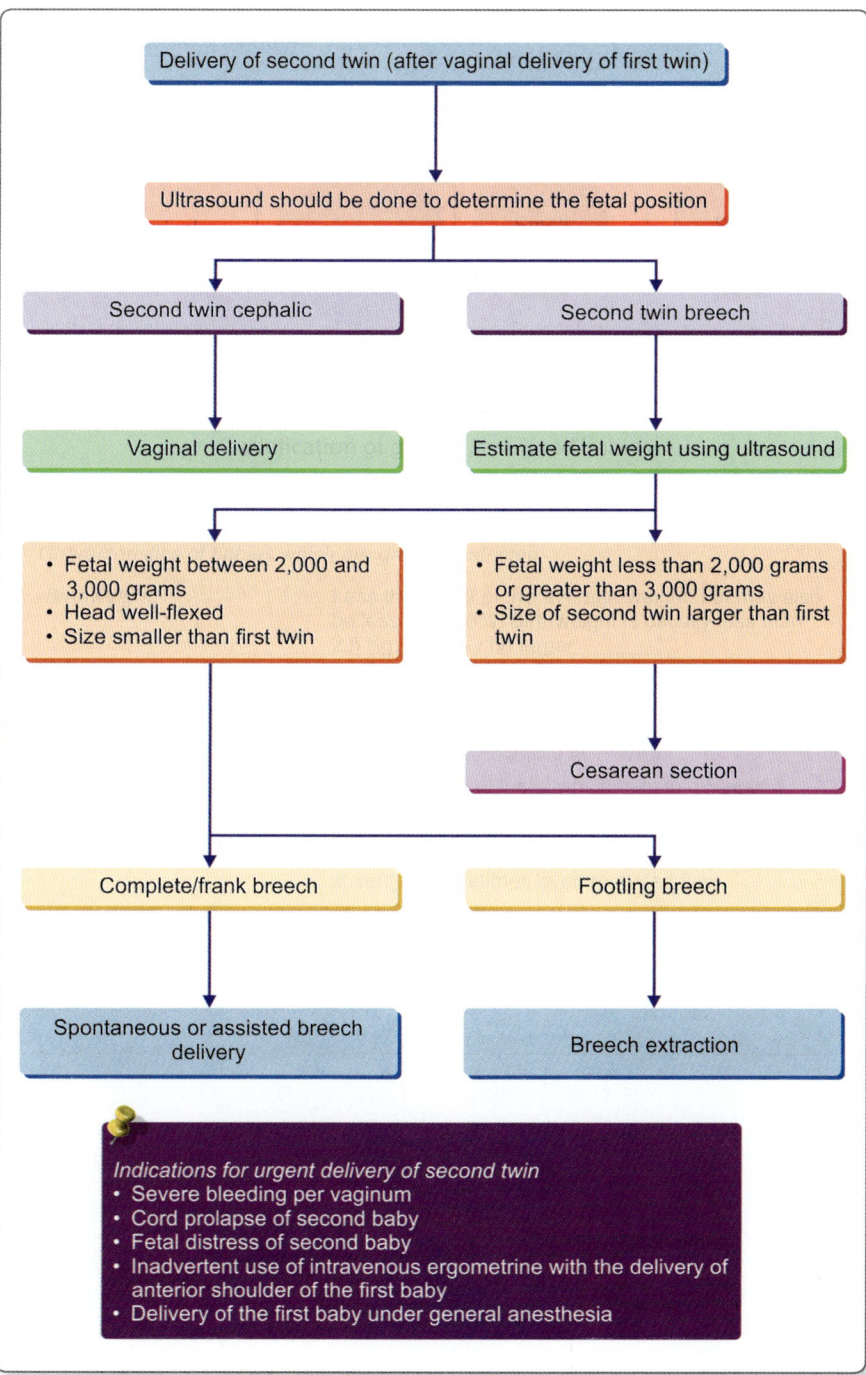

Flow Chart 7.2 Intrapartum management of second twin in longitudinal lie

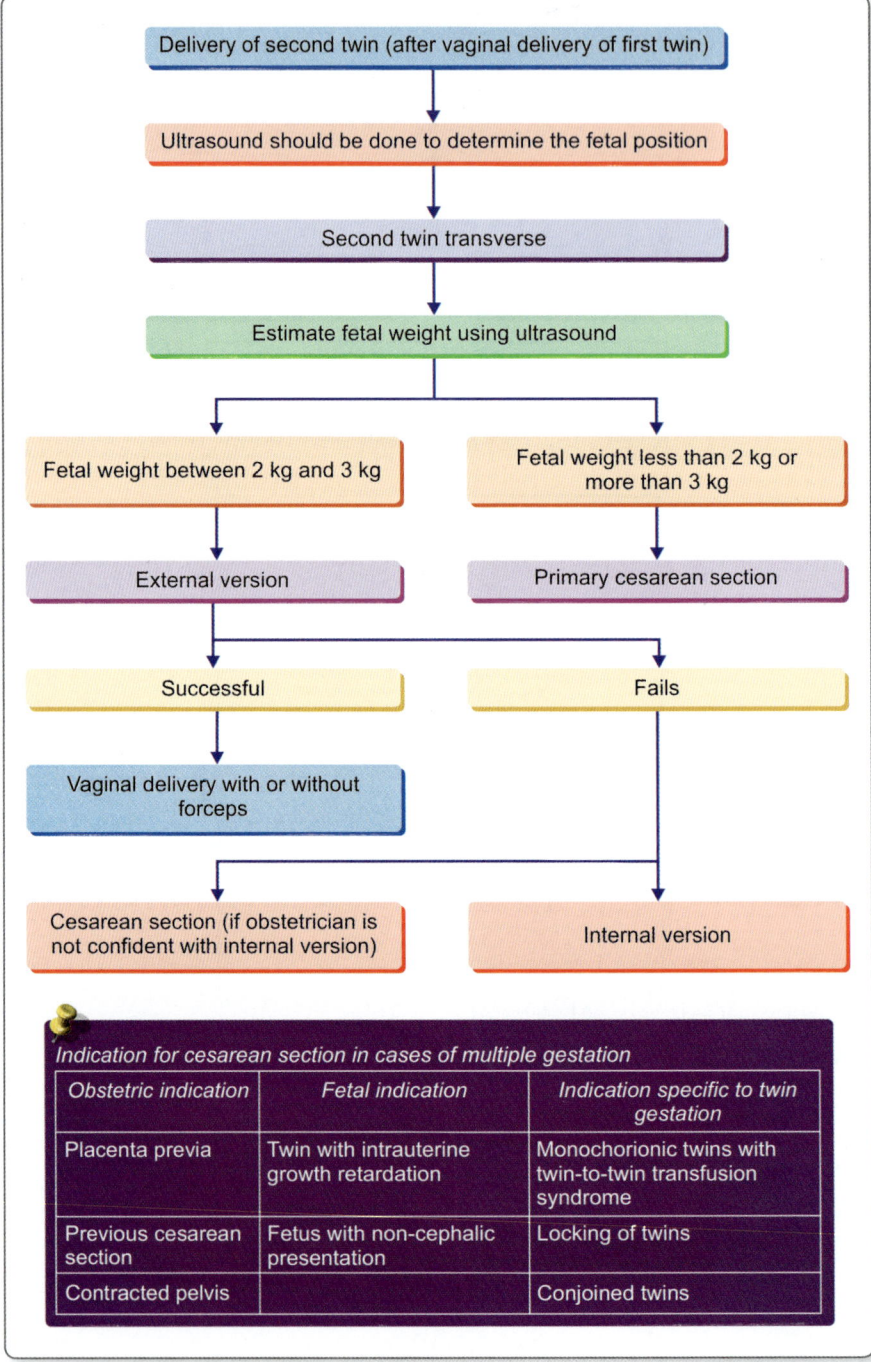

Flow Chart 7.3 Intrapartum management of second twin in transverse lie

8. Rh-Negative Pregnancy

ABO system and blood groups				
Blood group	RBC antigen	Plasma antibody	RBC choice	Plasma choice
A	A	Anti-B	A, O	A, AB
B	B	Anti-A	B, O	B, AB
AB	A, B	None	A, B, AB, O	AB
O	None	Anti-A, Anti-B	O	O, A, B, AB
Rh system and blood grouping				
Rh group	Rh antigen	Rh antibody	RBC choice	Plasma choice
Rh positive	D positive	None	Positive or negative	Either
Rh negative	D negative	Anti-D	Negative	Either

Two major classification systems for grouping blood, based on the presence of different of antigens: the "ABO system" and the "rhesus system"

Criteria for administration of second dose of anti-D immunoglobulins
- The baby born is Rh-positive
- Direct Coomb's test on the umbilical cord blood is negative
- The cross match between the anti-D immunoglobulins and mother's red cells is compatible

Criteria for administration of second dose of anti-D immunoglobulins to Rh-negative nonimmunized women

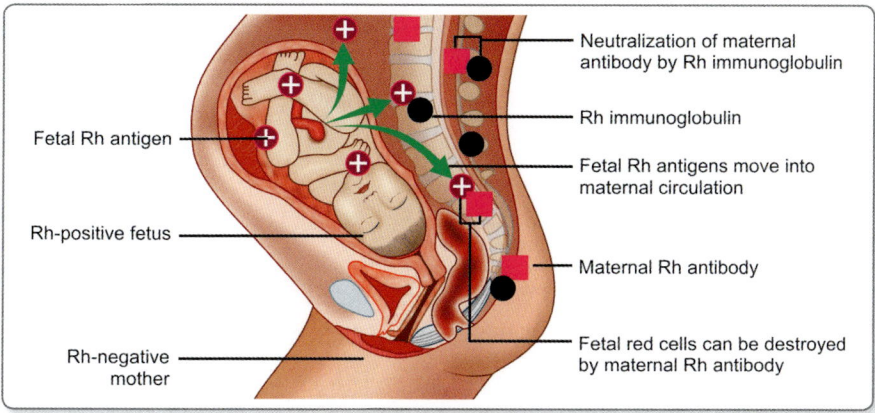

Mechanism of action of anti-D immunoglobulin's

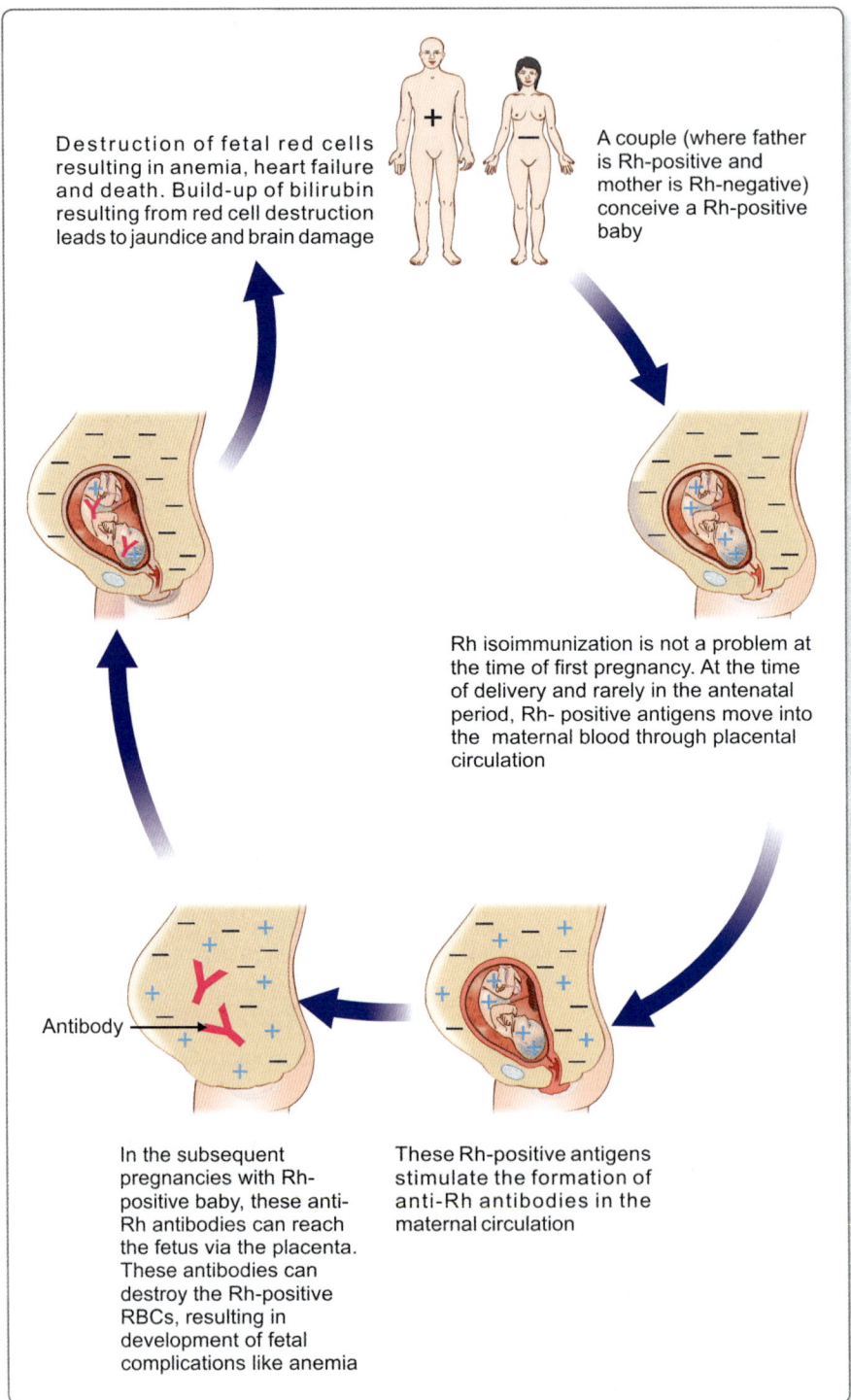

Flow Chart 8.1 Pathogenesis of Rh isoimmunization

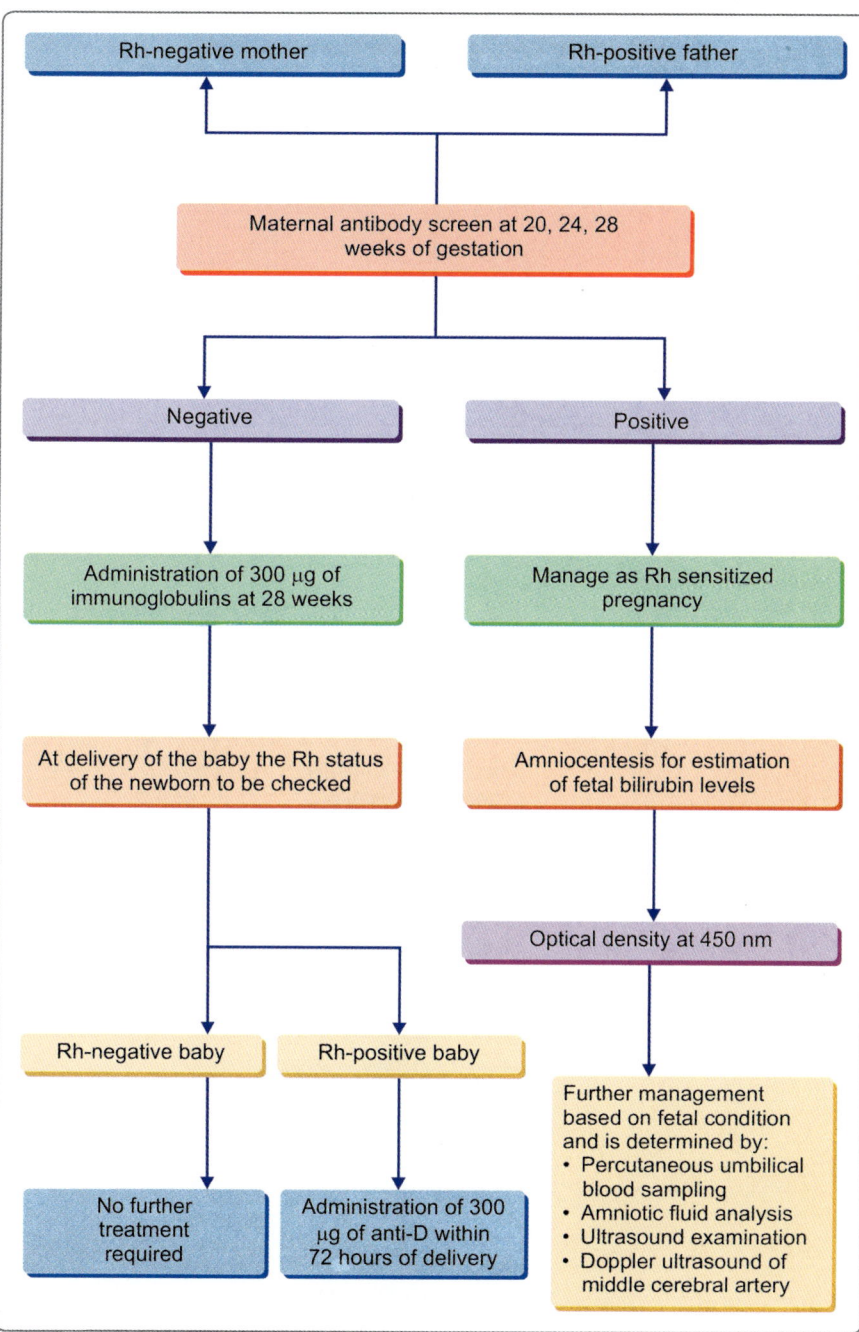

Flow Chart 8.2 Management of Rh negative nonimmunized women

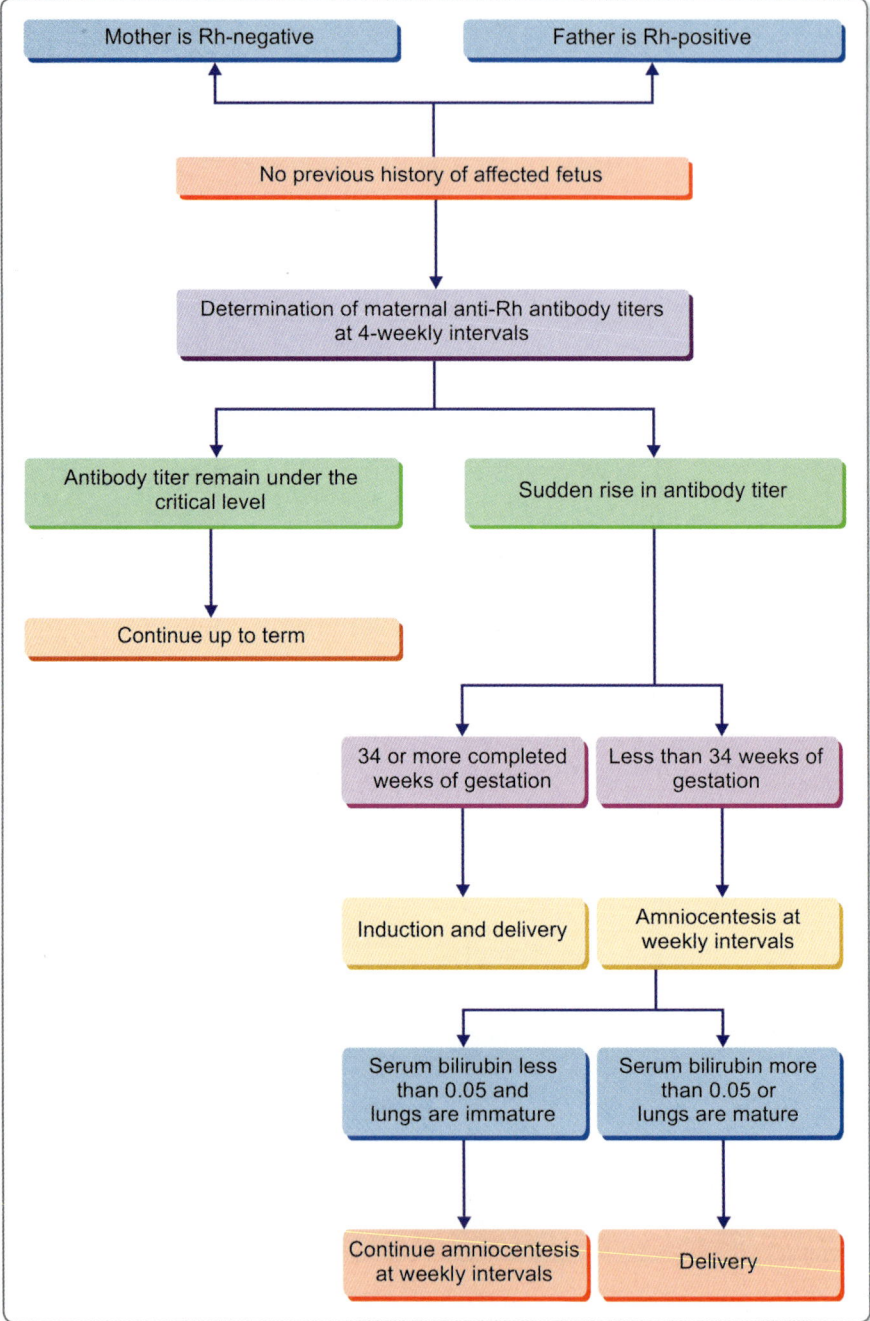

Flow Chart 8.3 Antenatal management of immunized Rh negative pregnancy with previous unaffected fetuses

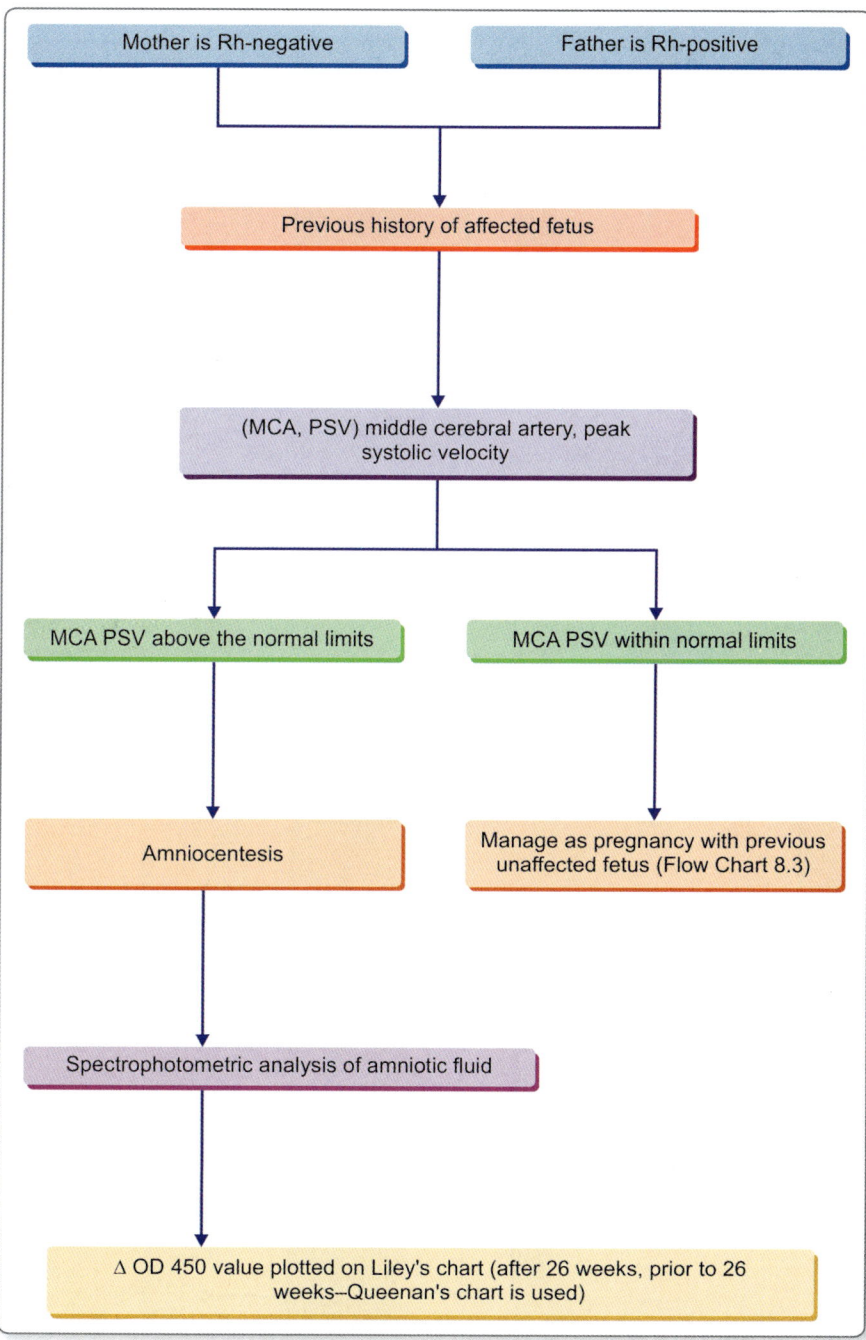

Flow Chart 8.4　Antenatal management of immunized Rh negative pregnancy with previous affected fetuses

Section 3 ❖ Pregnancy-Related Complications

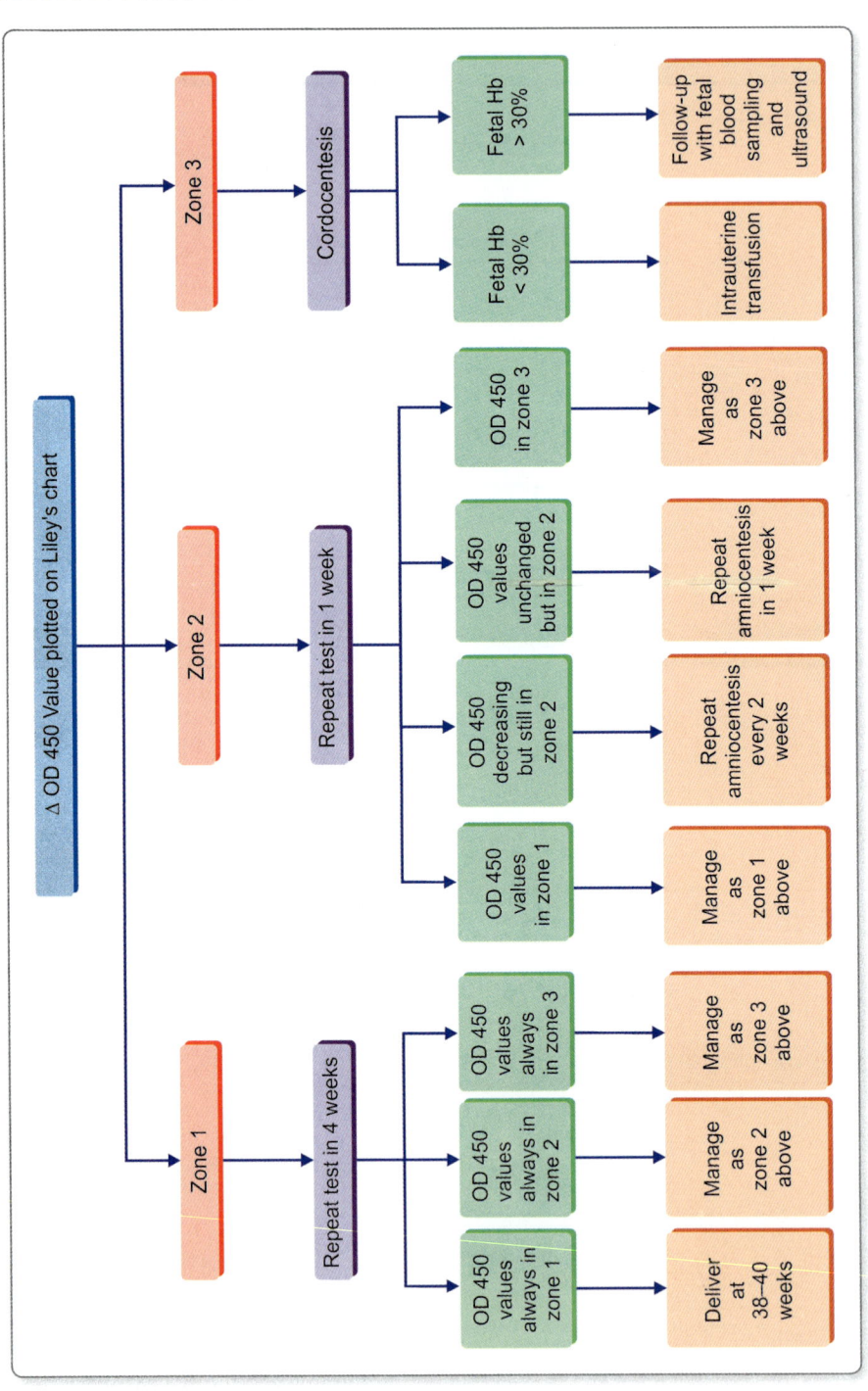

Flow Chart 8.5 Intrapartum management of immunized Rh negative pregnancy with previous affected fetuses

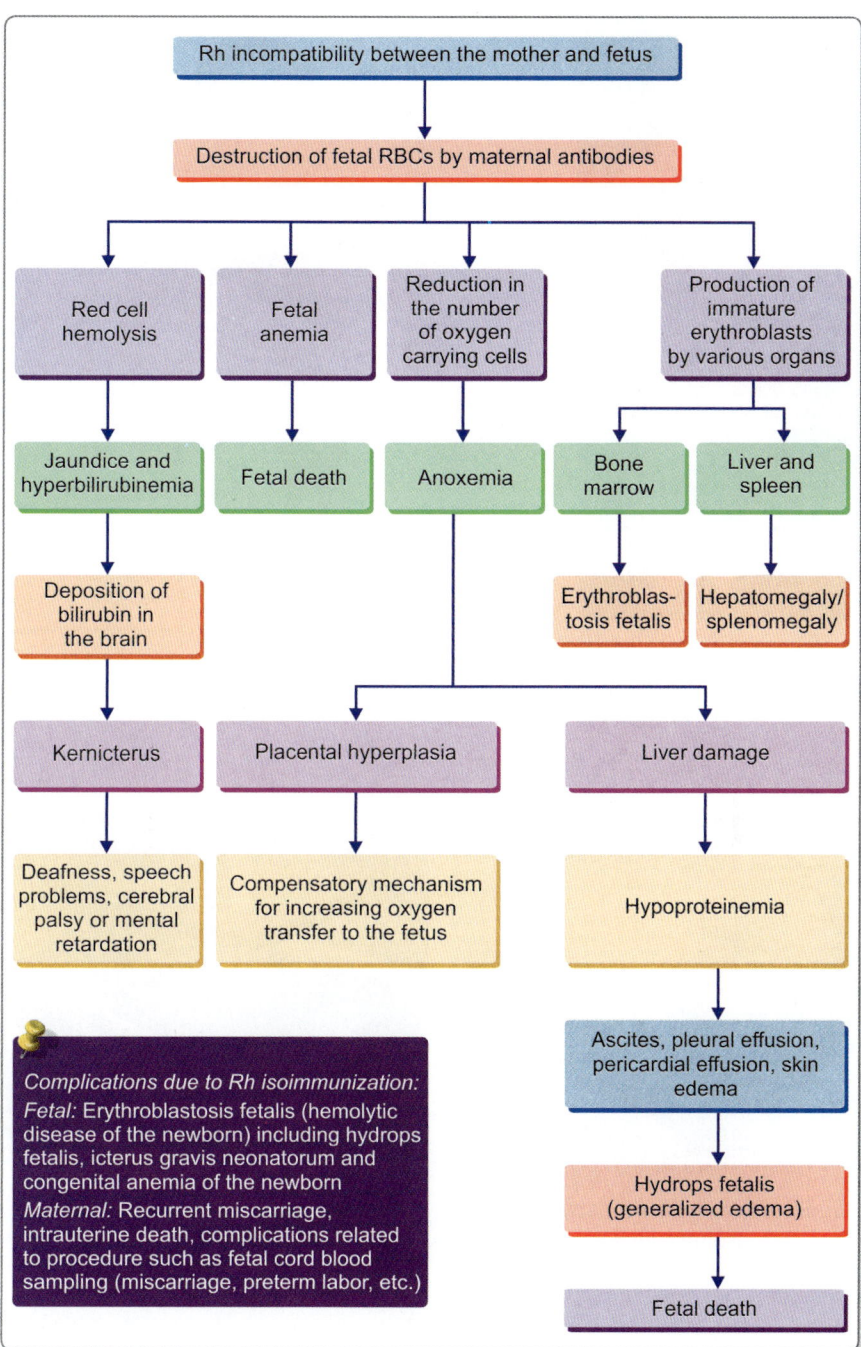

Flow Chart 8.6   Various fetal complications arising from Rh isoimmunization

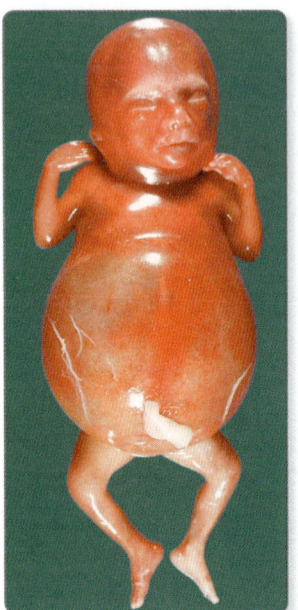
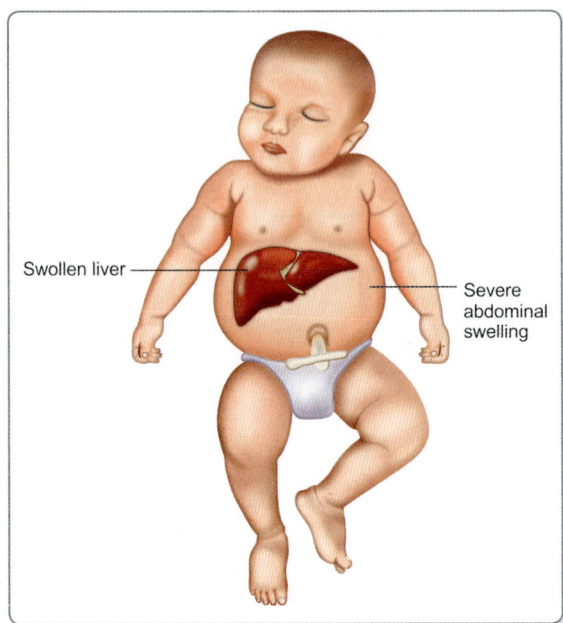

Hydrops fetalis associated with fetal ascites and skin edema

Diagrammatic representation of hydrops fetalis

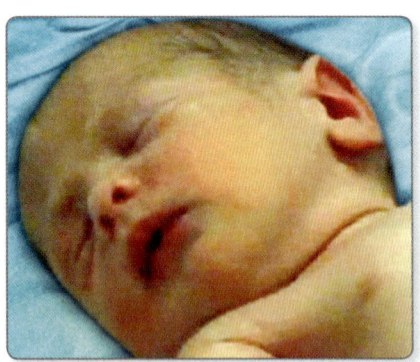
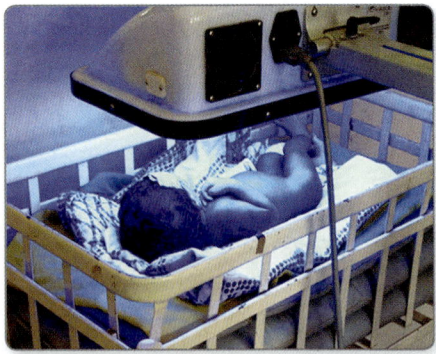

Jaundice in a newborn baby due to Rh isoimmunization

A newborn baby with mild degree of postnatal jaundice as a result of Rh isoimmunization being treated with phototherapy

9 Hydatidiform Mole

Hydatidiform mole (H. mole) belongs to a spectrum of disease known as gestational trophoblastic disease, resulting from overproduction of the chorionic tissue, which is normally supposed to develop into the placenta. H. mole can be considered as a neoplasm of trophoblastic tissue and involves both syncytiotrophoblast and cytotrophoblast

Definition of hydatidiform mole

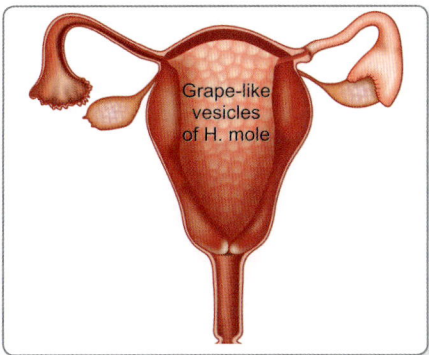

Grape-like vesicles of H.mole

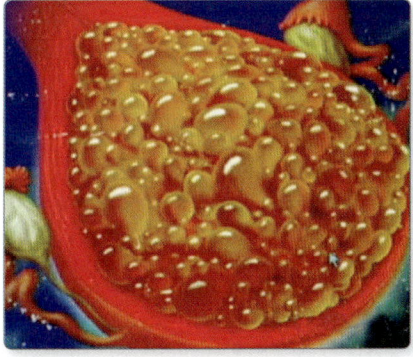

An artist's interpretation of H. mole

Classification of gestational trophoblastic disease
Benign forms (90%)
- Complete H. mole
- Partial H. mole

Malignant forms (10%)
Invasive mole
- Choriocarcinoma
- Placental site trophoblastic tumor
- Epithelioid trophoblastic tumor

Different types of gestational trophoblastic disease

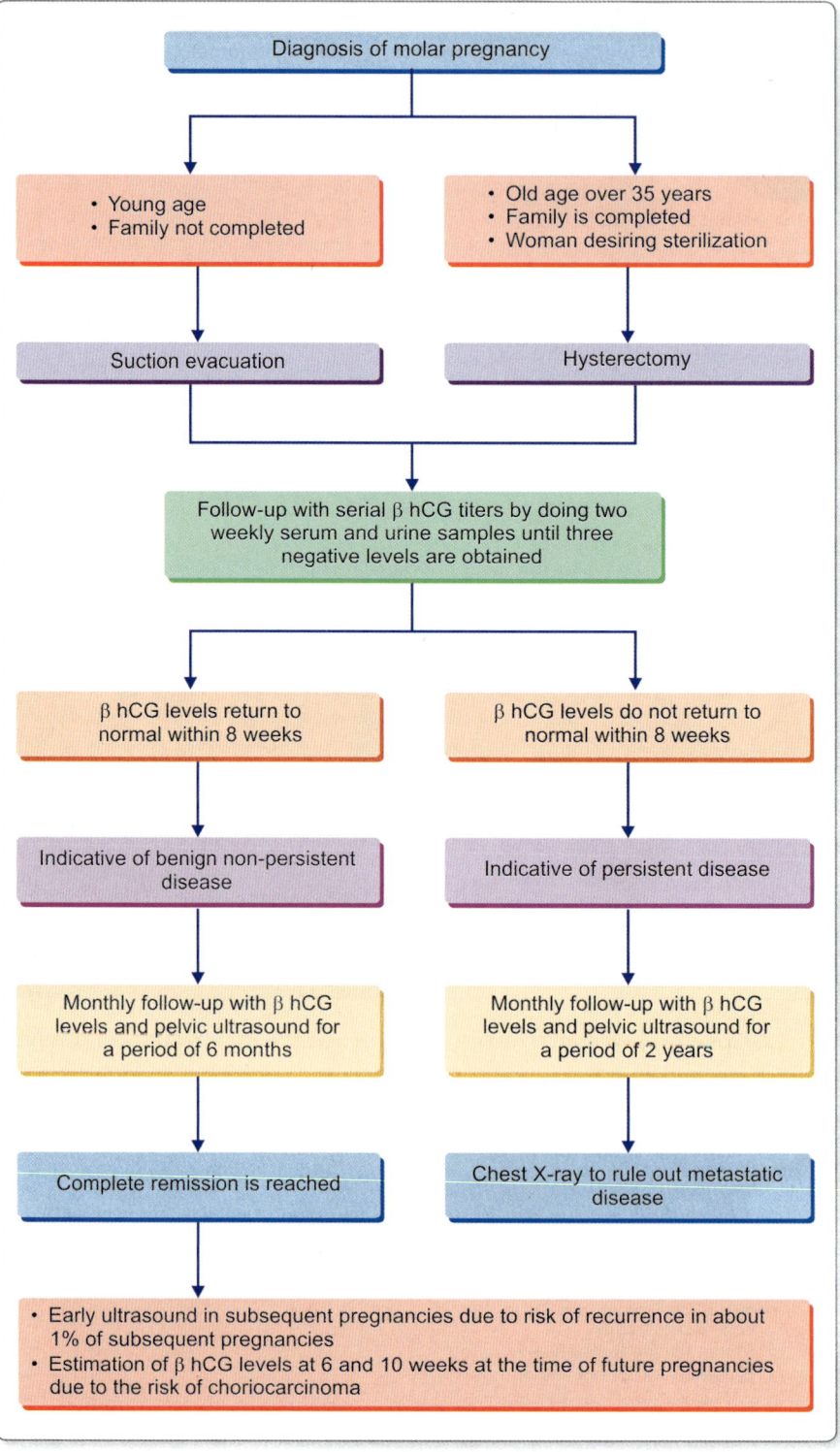

Flow Chart 9.1 Management of molar pregnancy

Comparison between complete and partial mole

Parameter under consideration	Complete mole	Partial mole
Cytogenetic studies	46XX karyotype	Triploid karyotype 69XXY
Pathophysiology	Duplication of the haploid sperm following fertilization of an "empty" ovum or dispermic fertilization of an "empty" ovum	These contain two sets of paternal haploid genes and one set of maternal haploid genes. They usually occur following dispermic fertilization of an ovum
Histopathological analysis	There is no evidence of fetal tissue	There may be an evidence of fetal tissue or red blood vessels
Invasive potential and propensity for malignant transformation	Persistent trophoblastic disease following uterine evacuation may develop in about 15% cases with a complete mole	Persistent trophoblastic disease may develop in less than 5% cases of partial mole

Comparative analysis of complete and partial mole

The classification system by the WHO and FIGO for classifying gestational trophoblastic tumors and treatment protocols

	Risk score			
Risk factor	0	1	2	4
Age (years)	< 40	≥ 40	–	–
Antecedent pregnancy	Mole	Abortion	Term	–
Interval (end of antecedent pregnancy to chemotherapy) in months	< 4	4–6	7–13	> 13
Human chorionic gonadotropin (IU/L)	$< 10^3$	$10^3–10^4$	$10^4–10^5$	$> 10^5$
Number of metastasis	0	1–4	5–8	> 8
Site of metastasis	Lung	Spleen, kidney	Gastrointestinal tract	Brain, liver
Largest tumor mass	–	3–5 cm	> 5 cm	–
Previous chemotherapy	–	–	Single drug	≥ 2 drugs

Gestational trophoblastic tumors and treatment protocols as classified by the WHO and FIGO

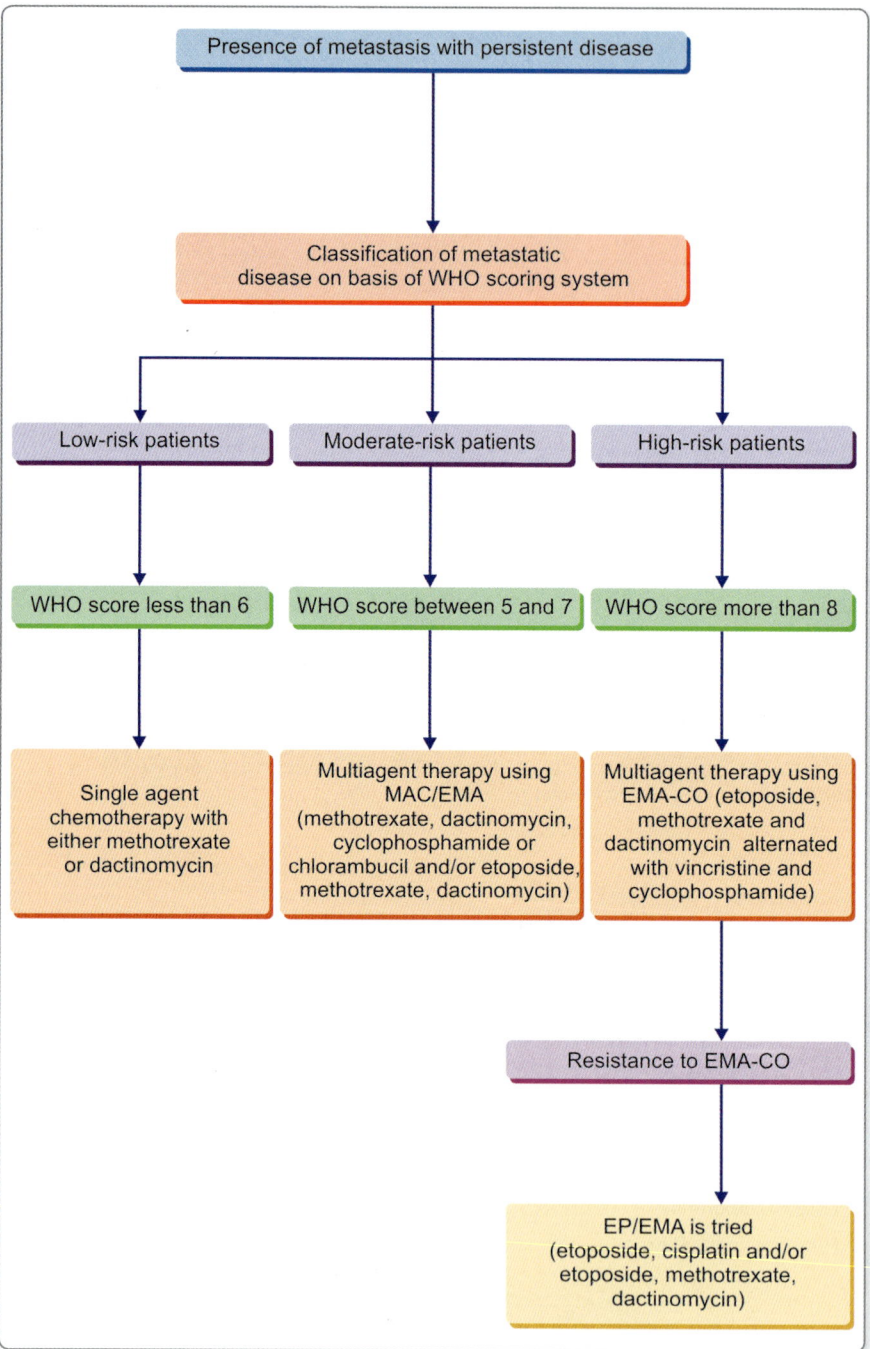

Flow Chart 9.2 Management of persistent disease with the presence of metastasis

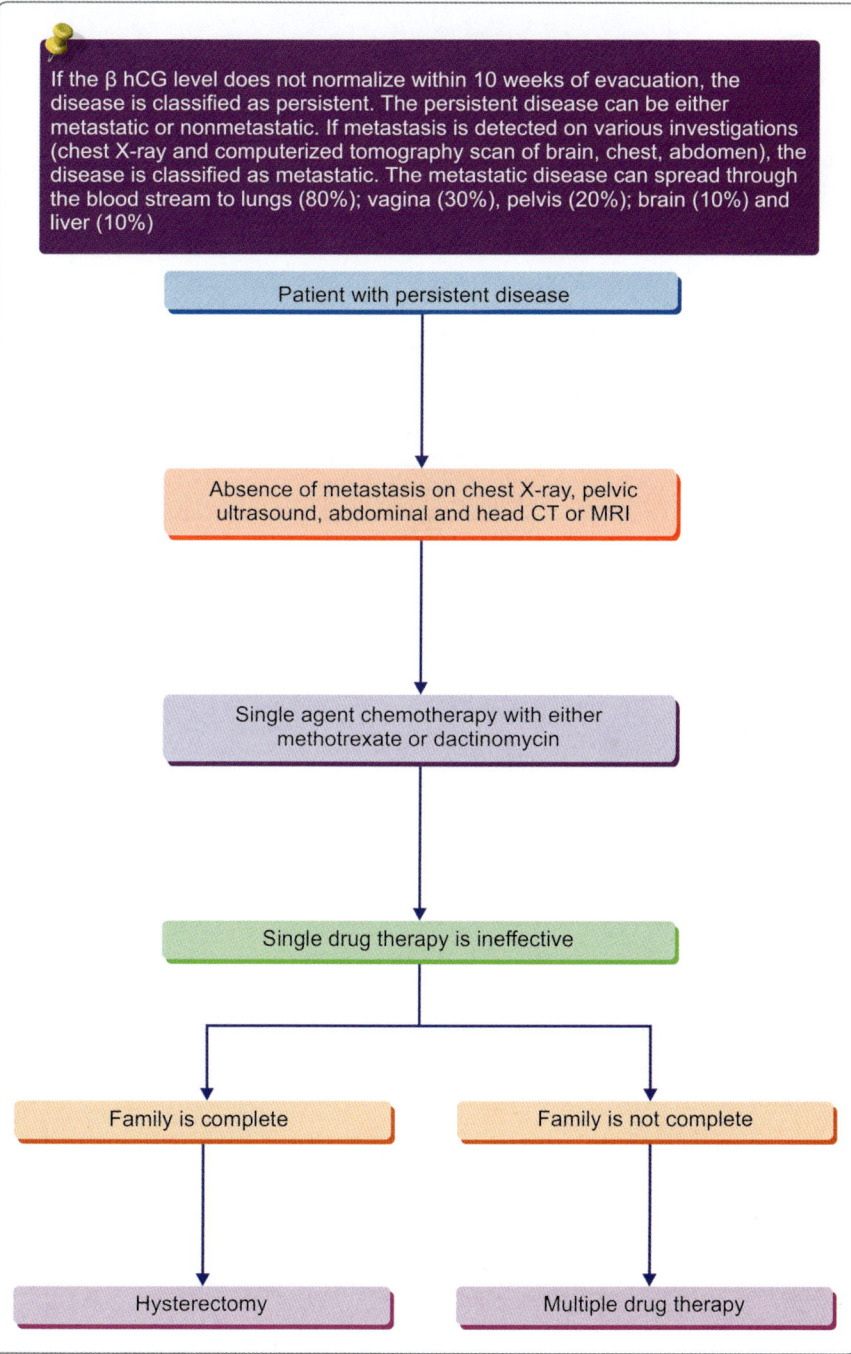

Flow Chart 9.3 Management of persistent disease with the absence of metastasis

10. Fetal Growth Restriction

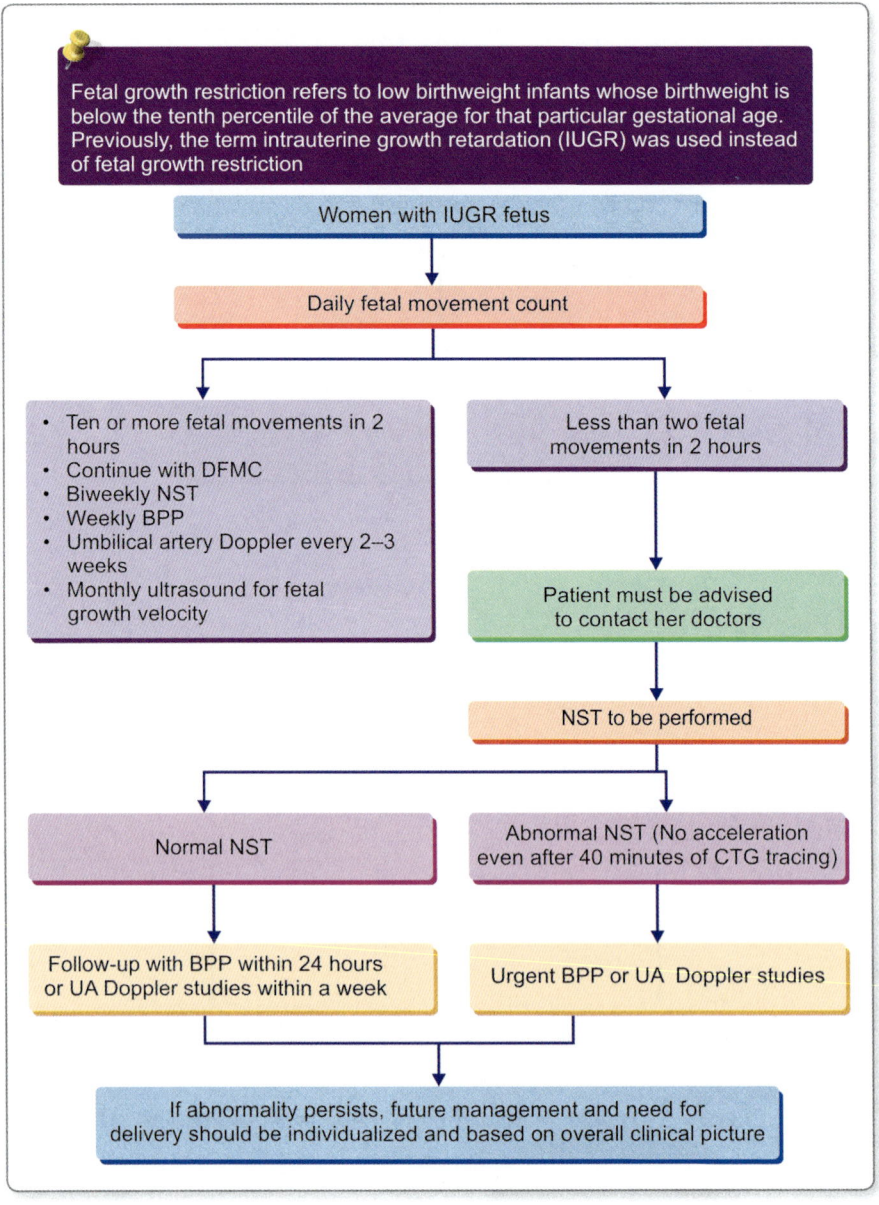

Flow Chart 10.1   Fetal surveillance in women with IUGR

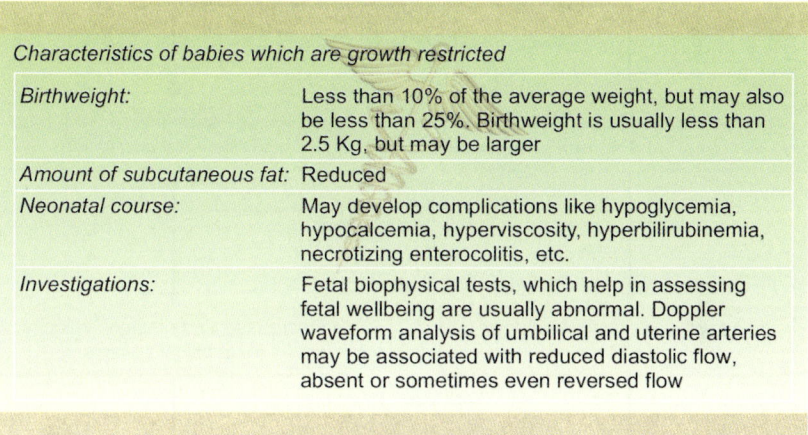

Classification of growth restricted babies

Characteristics of babies which are growth restricted	
Birthweight:	Less than 10% of the average weight, but may also be less than 25%. Birthweight is usually less than 2.5 Kg, but may be larger
Amount of subcutaneous fat:	Reduced
Neonatal course:	May develop complications like hypoglycemia, hypocalcemia, hyperviscosity, hyperbilirubinemia, necrotizing enterocolitis, etc.
Investigations:	Fetal biophysical tests, which help in assessing fetal wellbeing are usually abnormal. Doppler waveform analysis of umbilical and uterine arteries may be associated with reduced diastolic flow, absent or sometimes even reversed flow

Characteristics of IUGR babies

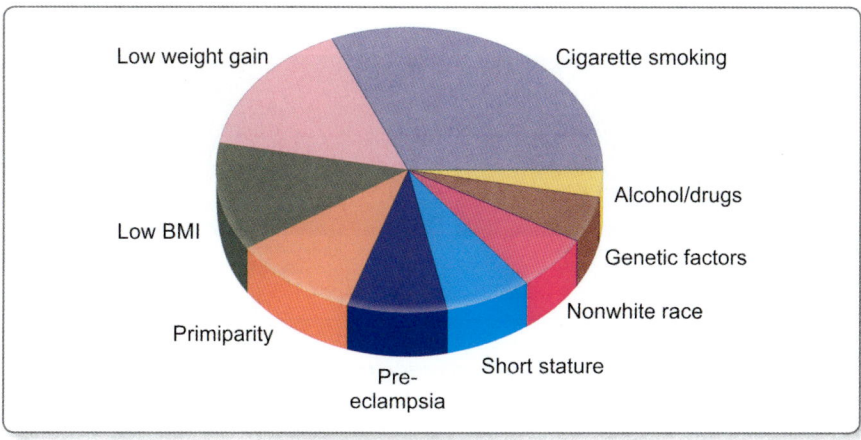

Causes of fetal growth retardation

Abbreviation: BMI, Body mass index

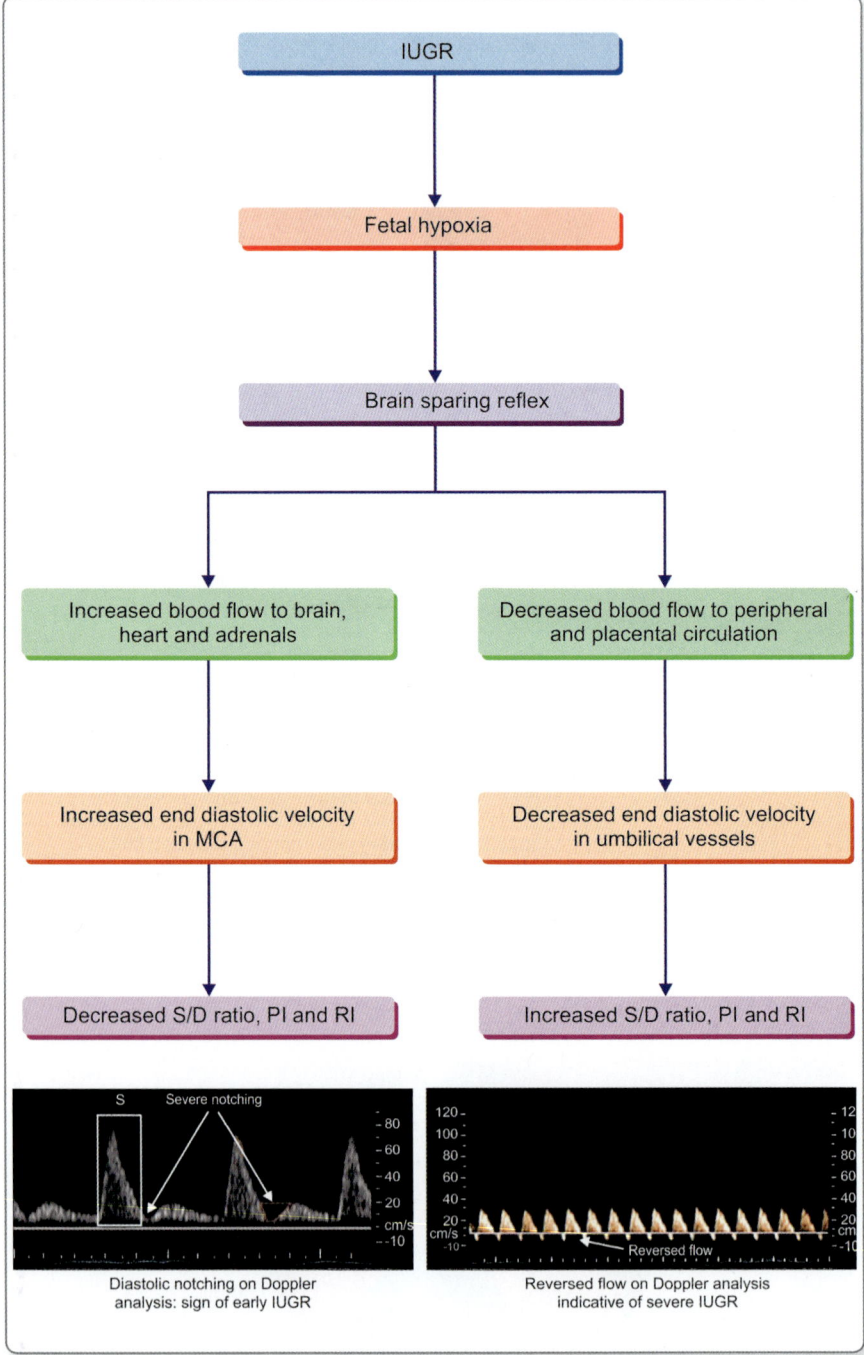

Flow Chart 10.2 Changes occurring in various Doppler velocity waveforms in IUGR fetuses

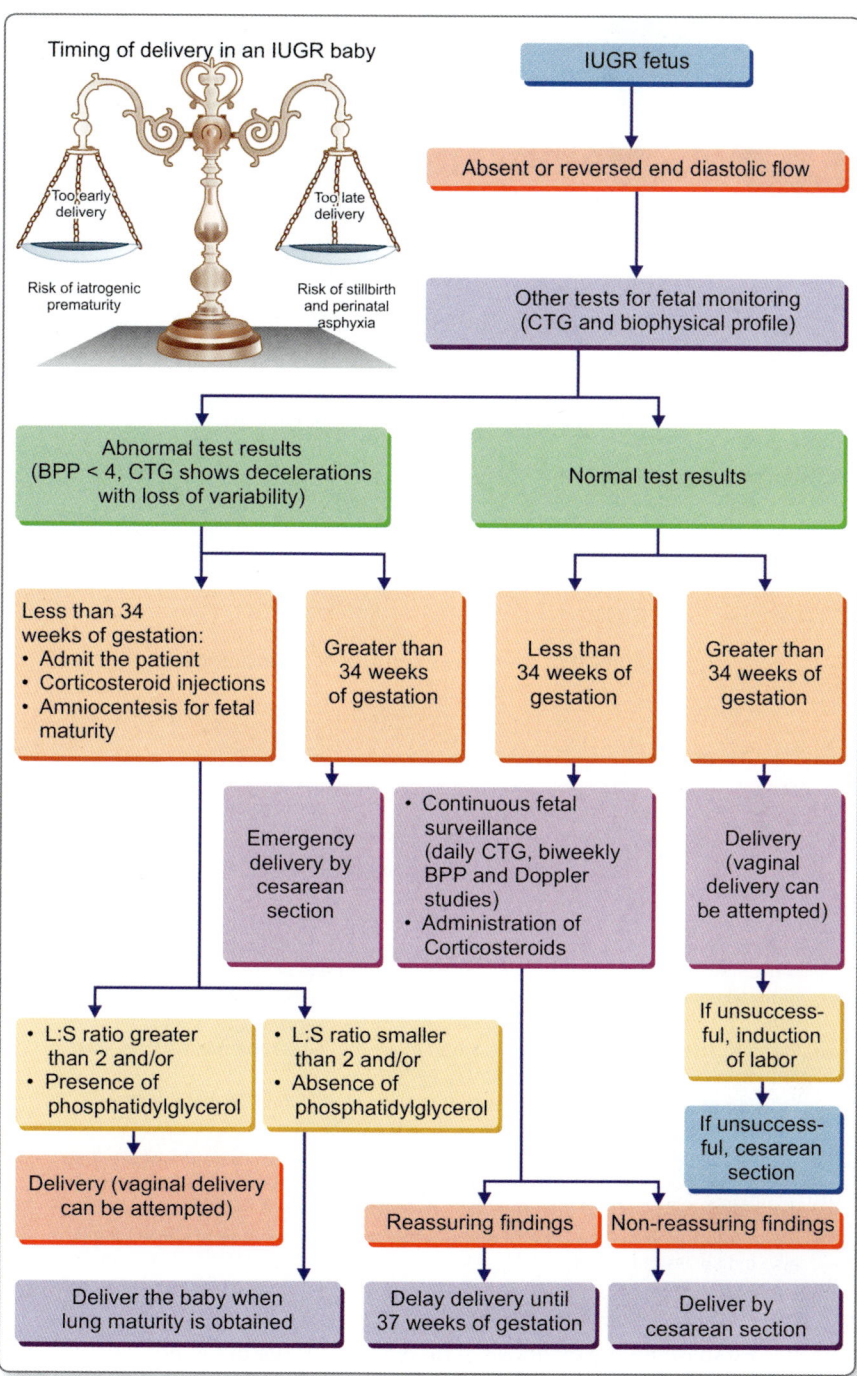

Flow Chart 10.3 Management plan for IUGR fetuses

 Premature Rupture of Membranes

Definition
Premature rupture of membranes (PROM) can be defined as spontaneous rupture of membranes (ROM), beyond 28 weeks of pregnancy, but before the onset of labor.

ROM occurring beyond 37 weeks of gestation, but before the onset of labor is known as term premature rupture of membranes. On the other hand, ROM occurring before 37 completed weeks of gestation, but before the onset of labor is called preterm PROM (PPROM). If the ROM is present for more than 24 hours before delivery, it is known as prolonged ROM

Definition of premature rupture of membranes

Diagnosis of premature rupture of membranes
The diagnosis of premature rupture of membranes can be confirmed by the following tests:
- *Nitrazine paper test:* The pH of the fluid collected from the vaginal fornix must be detected using litmus or nitrazine paper. In case of the presence of liquor (which is normally alkaline in nature, pH 7–7.5), the normally acidic vaginal pH (4.5–5.5) turns alkaline causing the color of the nitrazine paper to change from yellow to blue
- *Ferning:* The liquor smeared slide when examined under the microscope shows appearance of a characteristic ferning pattern
- *Staining of the centrifuged cells with 0.1% nile blue sulfate:* In case of PROM, there may be orange-blue discoloration of the cells
- *Intra-amniotic injection of lignocaine:* Presence of blue discoloration of the fluid emanating from cervical os, following injection of 2–3 mL of sterile solution of the dye indigo carmine into the amniotic cavity is indicative of PROM
- *Alpha-fetoproteins:* Presence of alpha-fetoproteins in the vaginal secretions is also indicative of PROM

Establishing the diagnosis of premature rupture of membranes

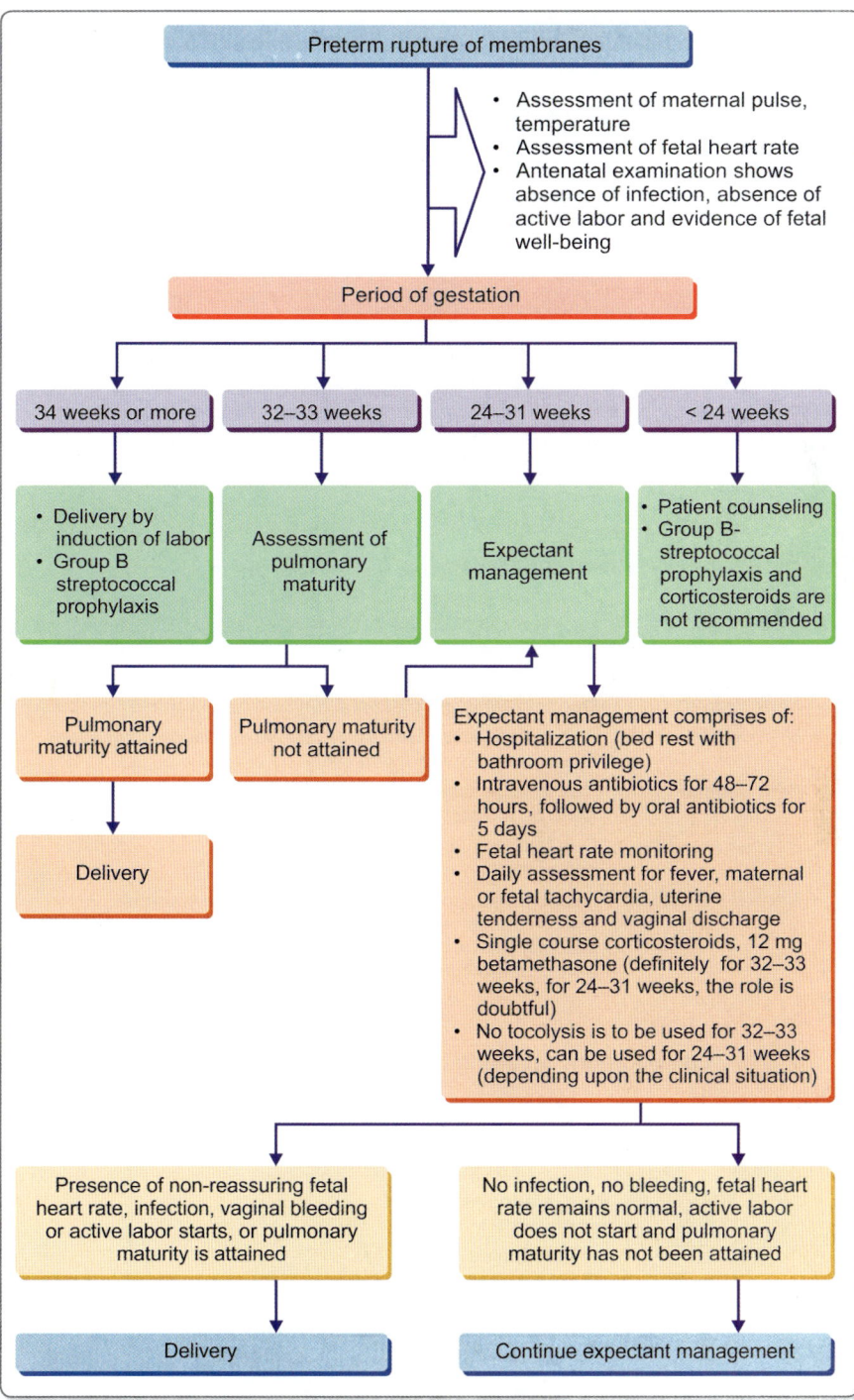

Flow Chart 11.1 Management of premature rupture of membranes

12 Post-Term Pregnancy

Definition
Post-term or postmature pregnancy can be defined as any pregnancy continuing beyond 2 weeks of the expected date of delivery (> 294 days). Prolonged labor can be expected in these cases due to a large baby and poor molding of the fetal head

Definition and course of post-term pregnancy

Complications of post-term pregnancy
- **Fetal distress:** Due to diminished placental function and oligohydramnios
- **Macrosomia:** This is associated with an increased incidence of shoulder dystocia and operative delivery
- **Birth trauma:** Due to large size of the baby and nonmolding of fetal head as a result of hardening of skull bones
- **Respiratory distress:** Due to chemical pneumonitis, atelectasis and pulmonary hypertension
- **Neonatal problems:** Hypothermia, poor subcutaneous fat, hypoglycemia, hypocalcemia, and increased incidence of injuries such as brachial plexus injuries. These result in an increased perinatal mortality and morbidity

Complications occurring due to post-term pregnancy

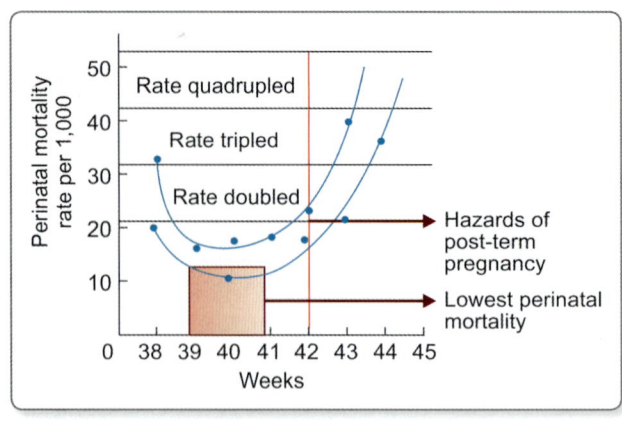

Consequences of a post-term pregnancy on perinatal outcomes

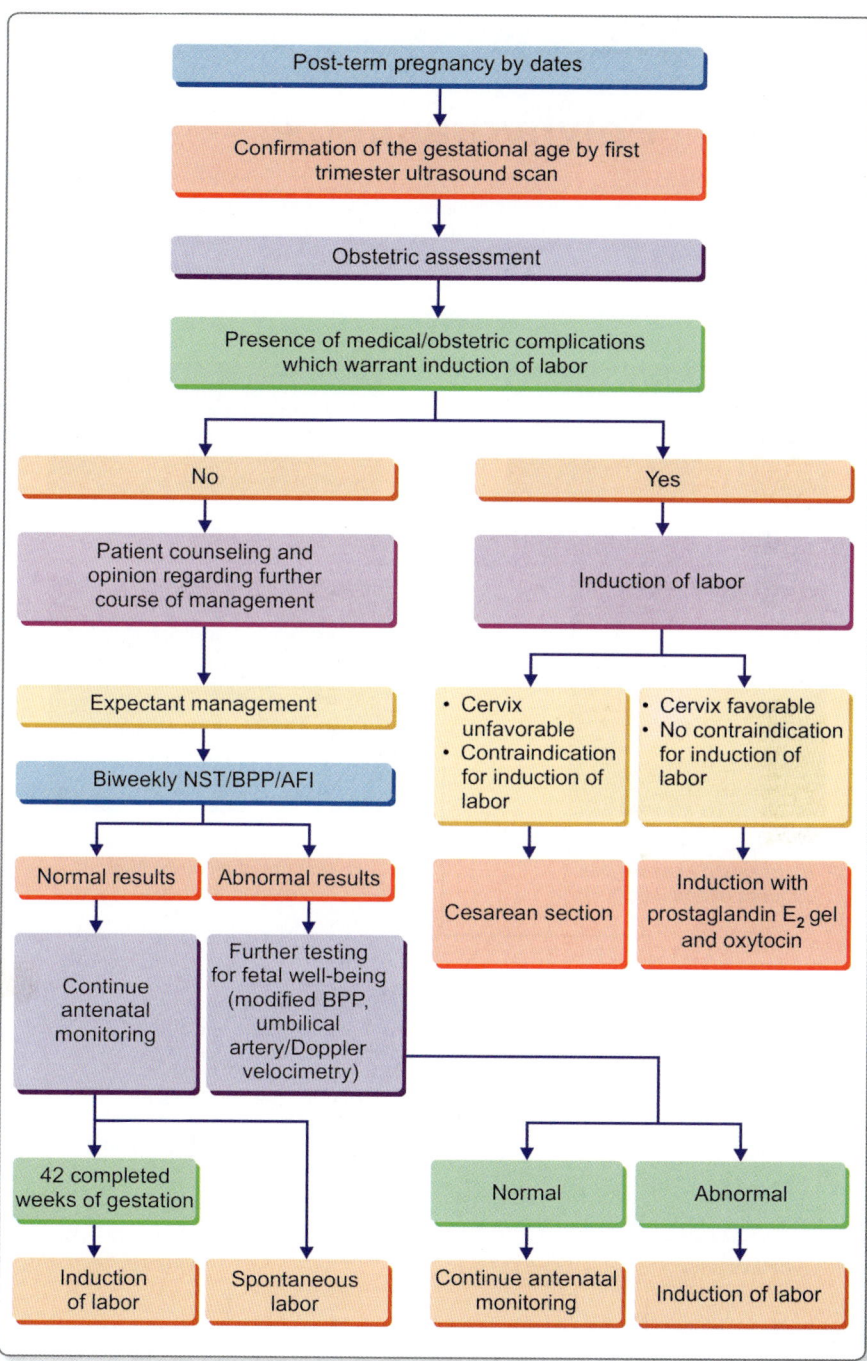

Flow Chart 12.1 Management of post-term pregnancies

13 Polyhydramnios

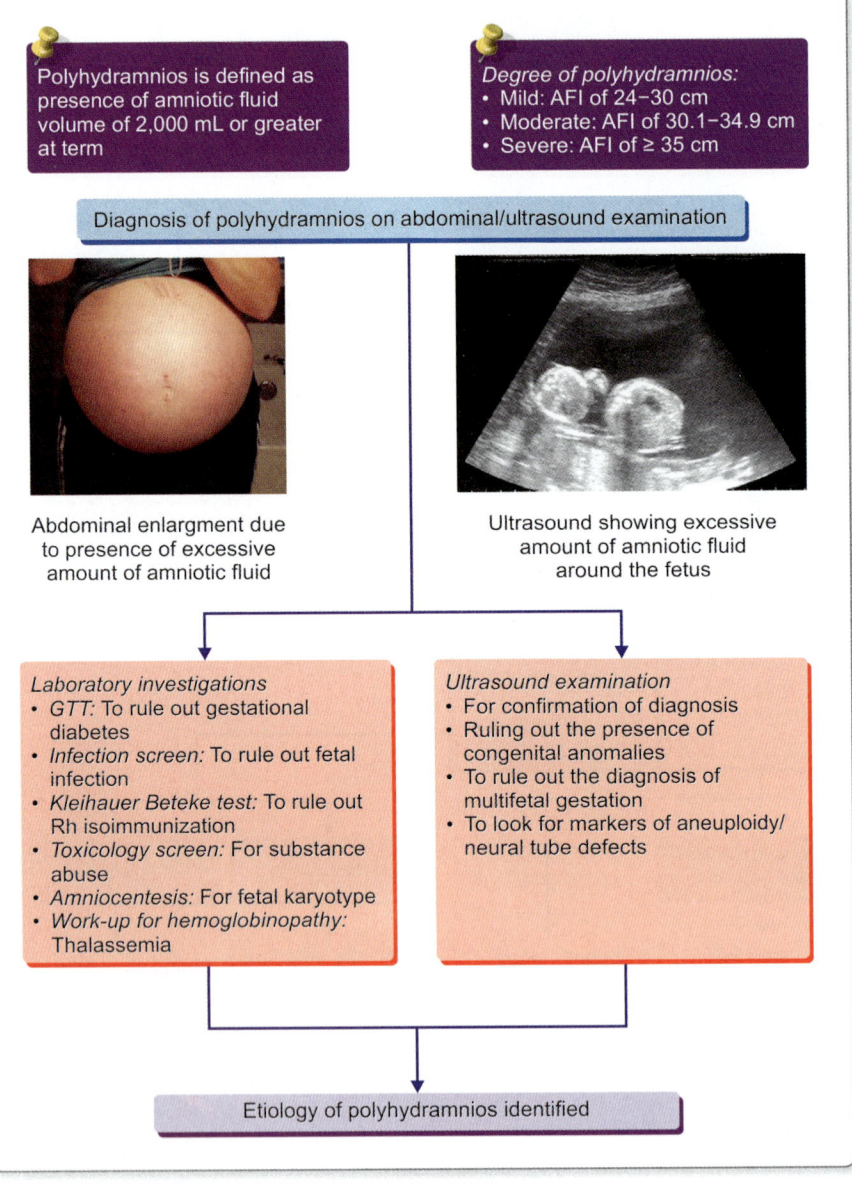

Flow Chart 13.1 Diagnosis of polyhydramnios with help of various tests

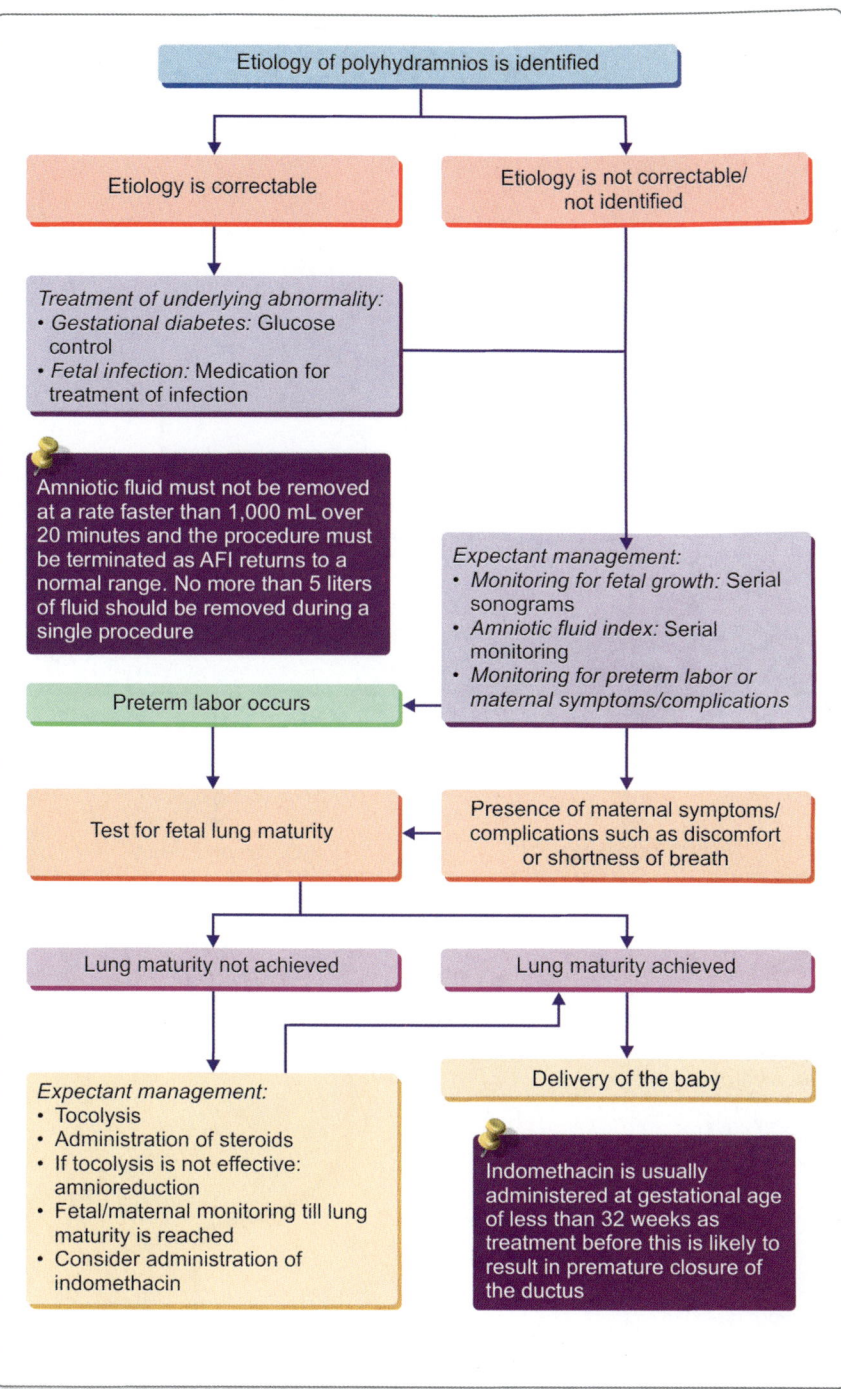

Flow Chart 13.2 Management of patient with polyhydramnios

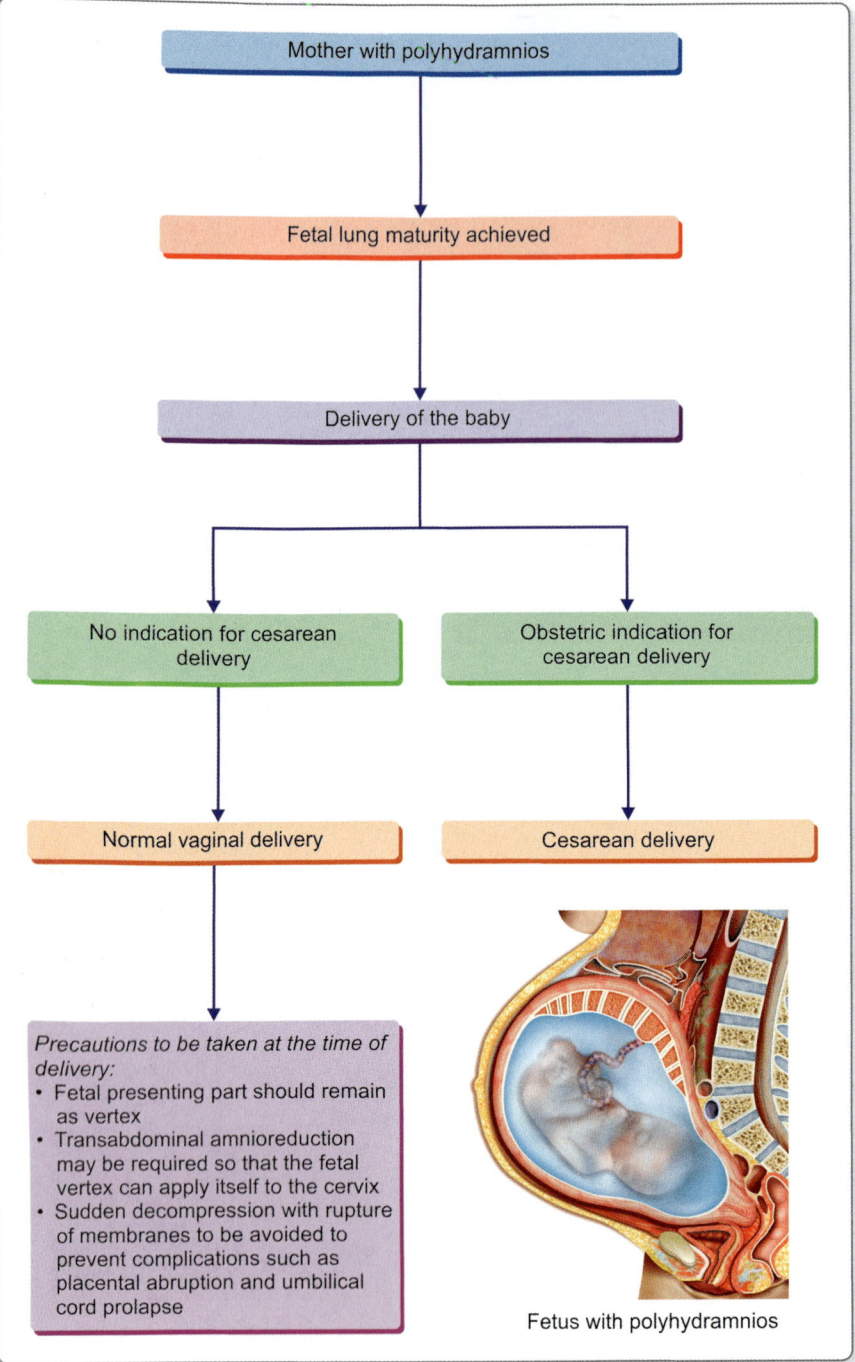

Flow Chart 13.3   Mode of delivery in a patient with polyhydramnios

14 Urogenital Fistula Due to Obstructed Labor

Definition
Urogenital fistula (UGF) can be defined as an abnormal communication tract (lined with epithelium) between the genital tract and the urinary tract or the alimentary tract or both. UGFs can be classified as follows:
- Urethrovaginal
- Vesical fistula (vesicovaginal fistula or vesicocervical)
- Ureterovaginal
- Rectovaginal

Definition and types of urogenital fistulas

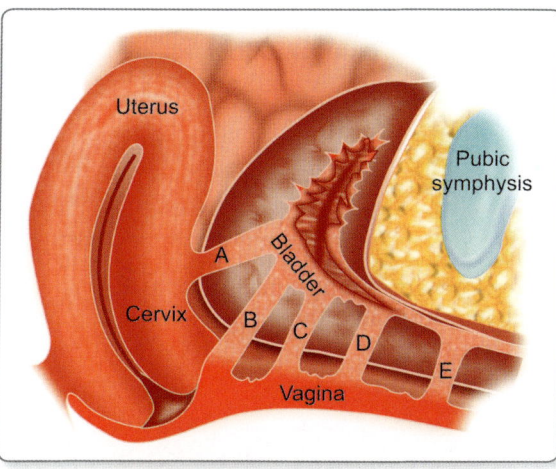

Types of genitourinary fistulas (A) uterovesical fistula; (B) vesicocervical fistula; (C) midvaginal VVF; (D) VVF involving the bladder neck; (E) urethrovaginal fistula

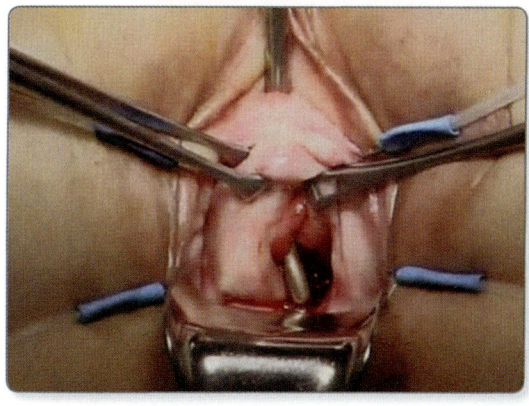

A dilator feing passed through the fistula tract in a patient with VVF undergoing surgery

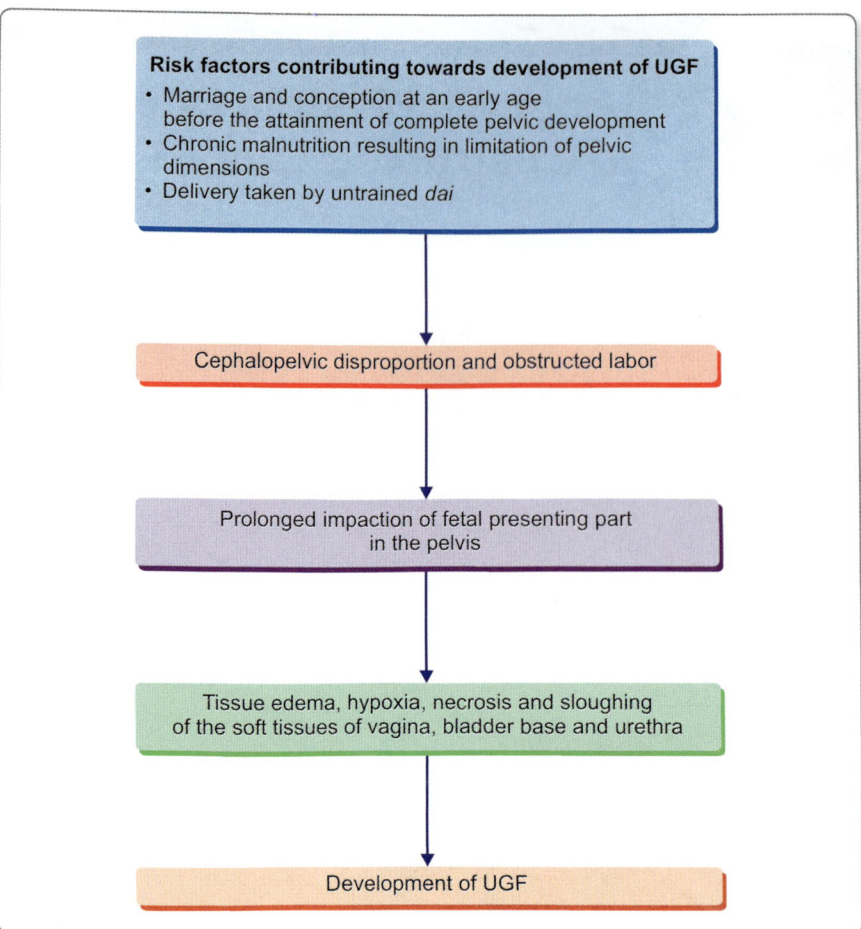

Flow Chart 14.1 Development of urogenital fistulas as a result of obstructed labor

A few clinical pointers related to genitourinary fistulae
- The most common type of fistula in the developing countries is VVF at the bladder neck region following difficult childbirth. Such a woman is often short statured with a contracted pelvis
- The uncontrolled continuous leakage of urine into the vagina is the hallmark symptom of patients with UGFs
- Prior to undertaking surgery, urine sample must be collected by catheterization and must be submitted for culture and sensitivity. Any infection must be treated prior to surgery
- At the time of surgery, routine excision of the fistula tract is not mandatory
- Successful fistula repair requires adequate dissection and mobilization of tissues, meticulous hemostasis and reapproximation under minimal tension

Clinical highlights related to genitourinary fistulas

15 Miscarriage

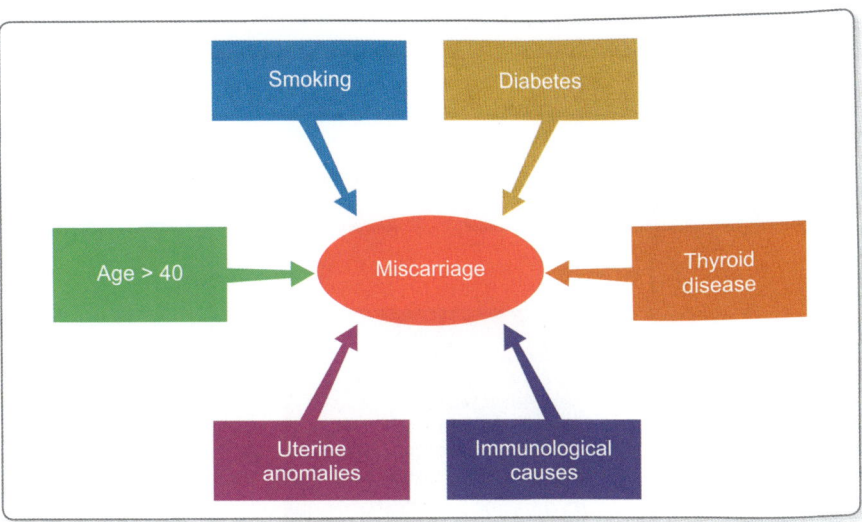

Various causes of miscarriage

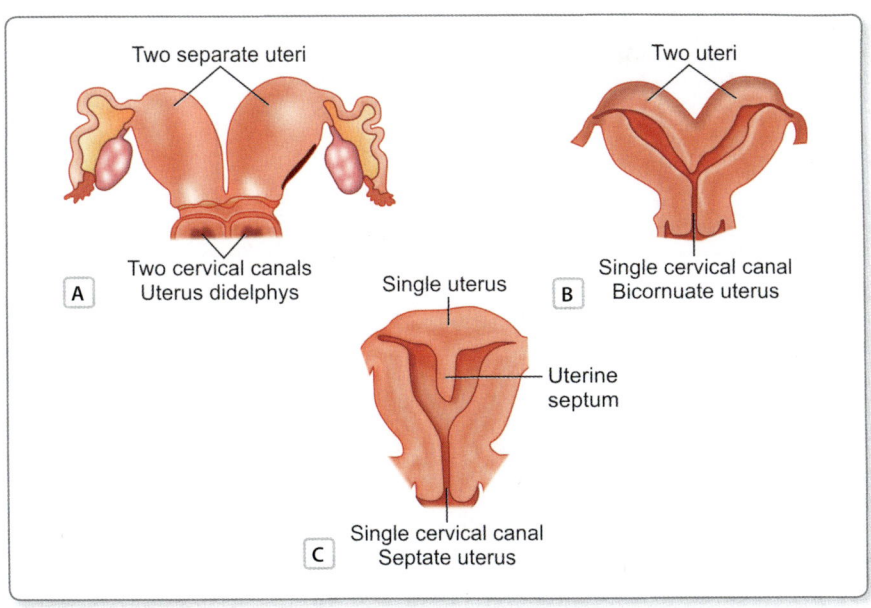

Various uterine anomalies as a cause of recurrent miscarriage: (A) uterus diadelphys; (B) bicornuate uterus; (C) septate uterus

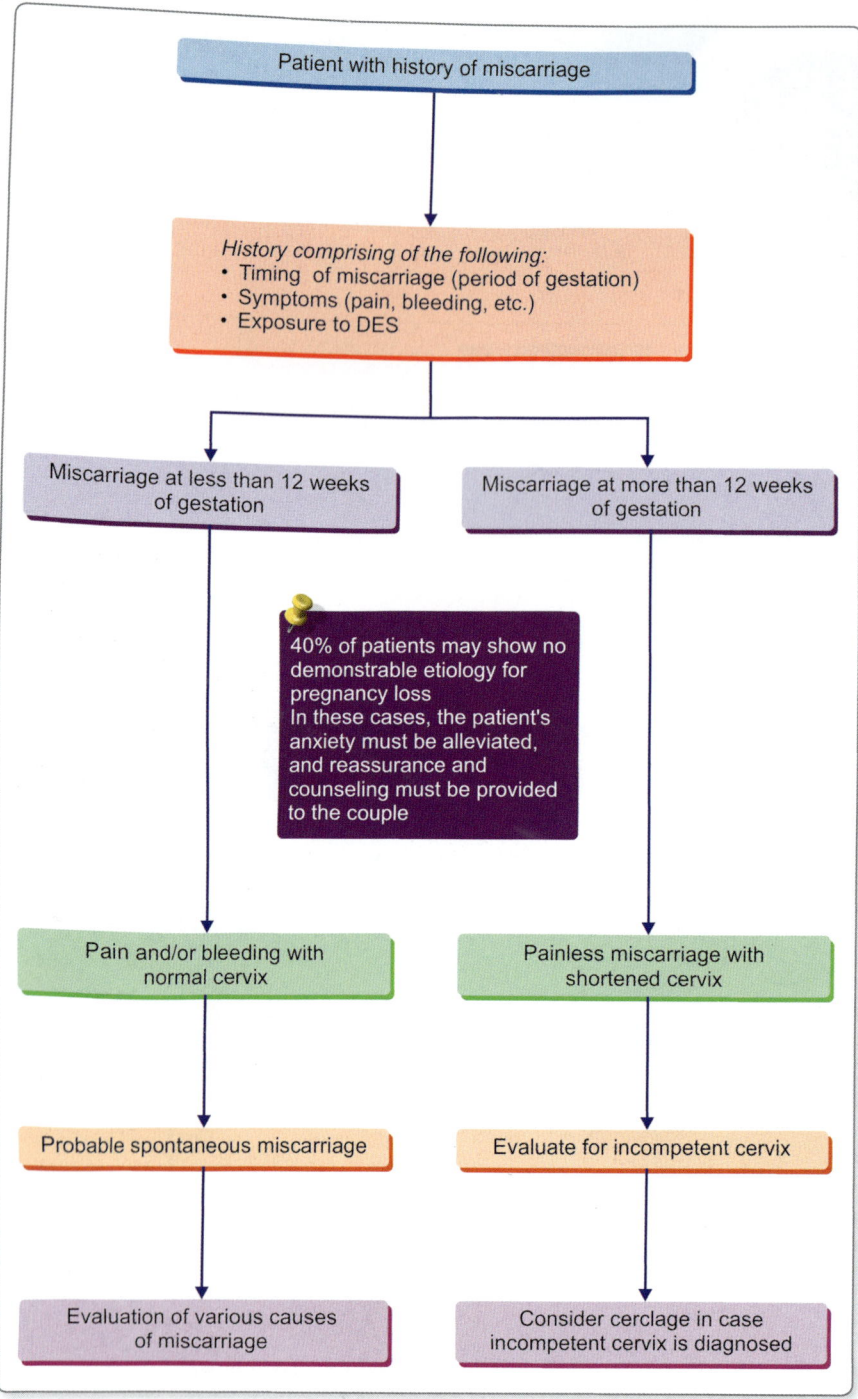

Flow Chart 15.1 Evaluation of a patient with miscarriage

15 Miscarriage

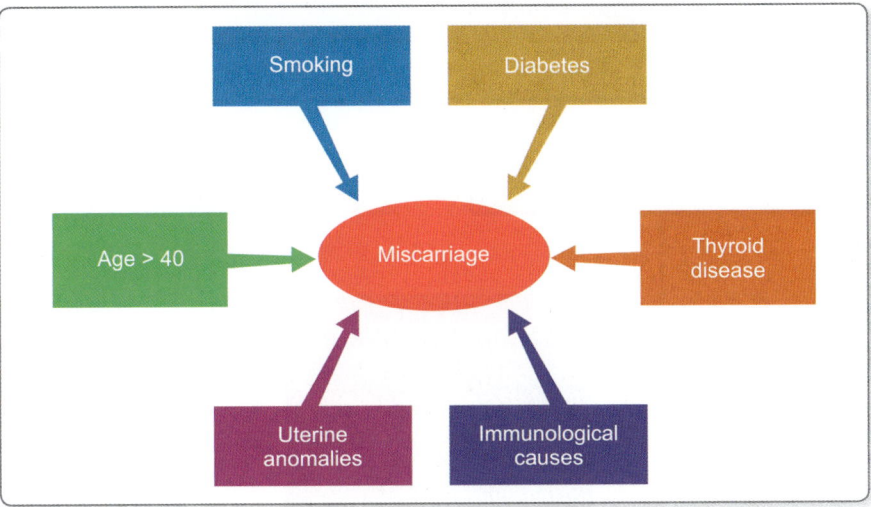

Various causes of miscarriage

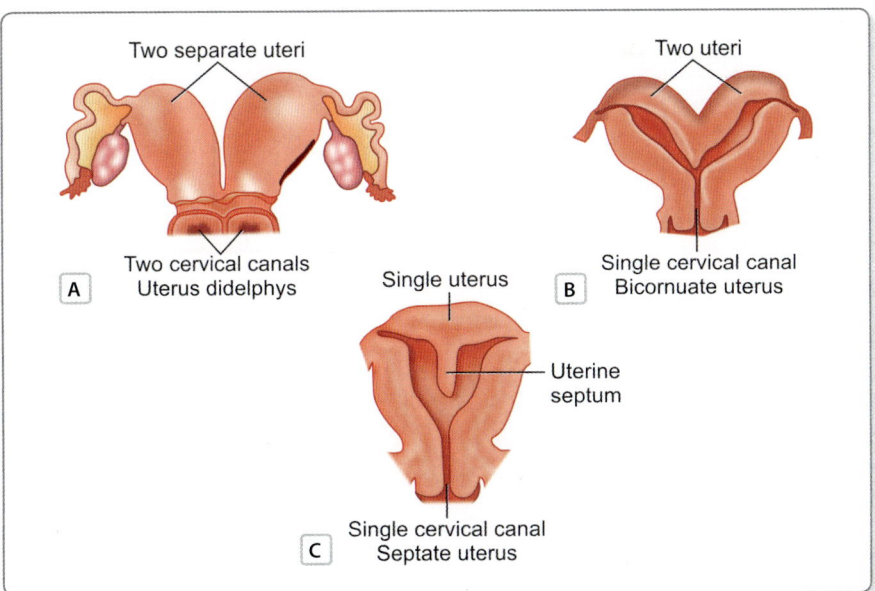

Various uterine anomalies as a cause of recurrent miscarriage: (A) uterus diadelphys; (B) bicornuate uterus; (C) septate uterus

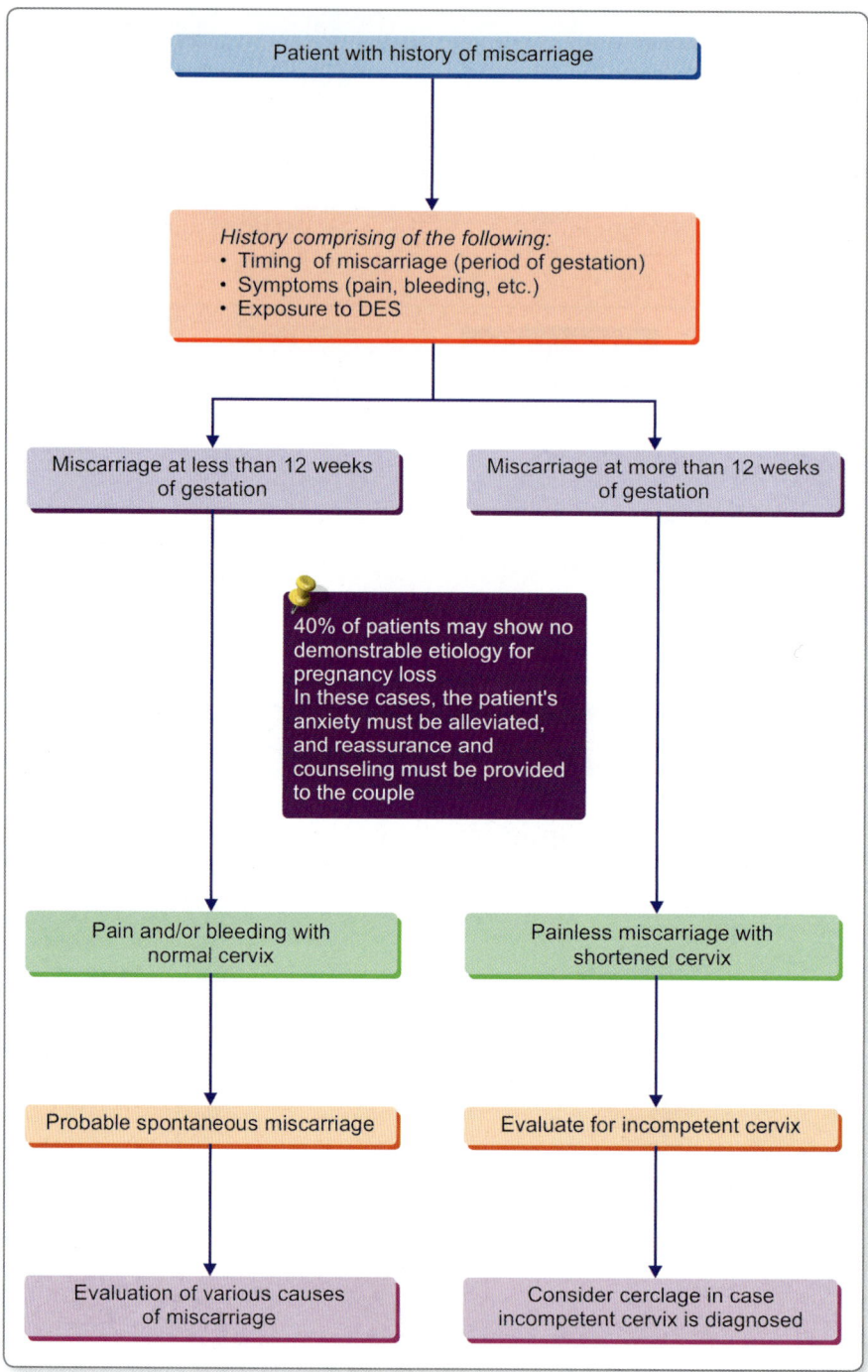

Flow Chart 15.1   Evaluation of a patient with miscarriage

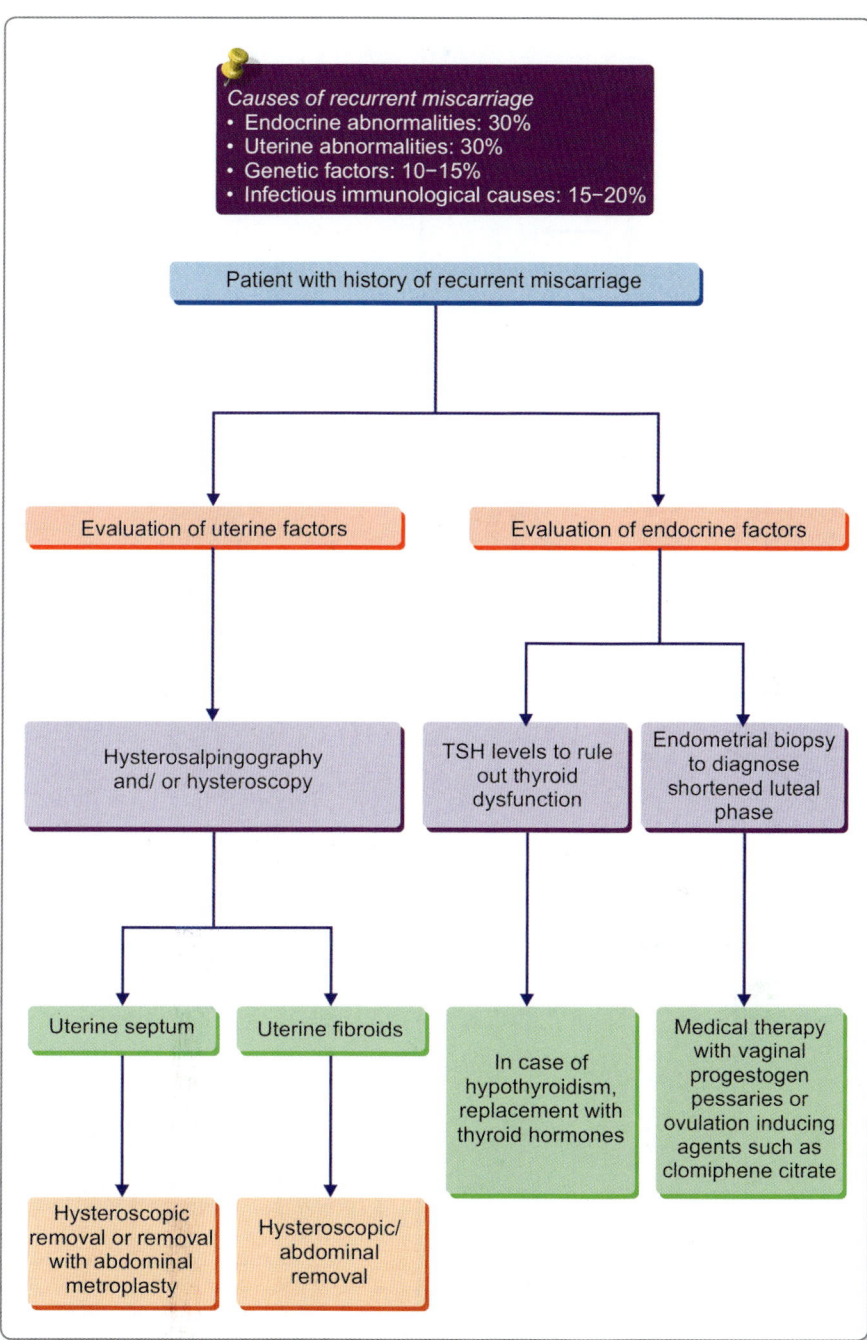

Flow Chart 15.2 Initial evaluation in cases of recurrent miscarriage

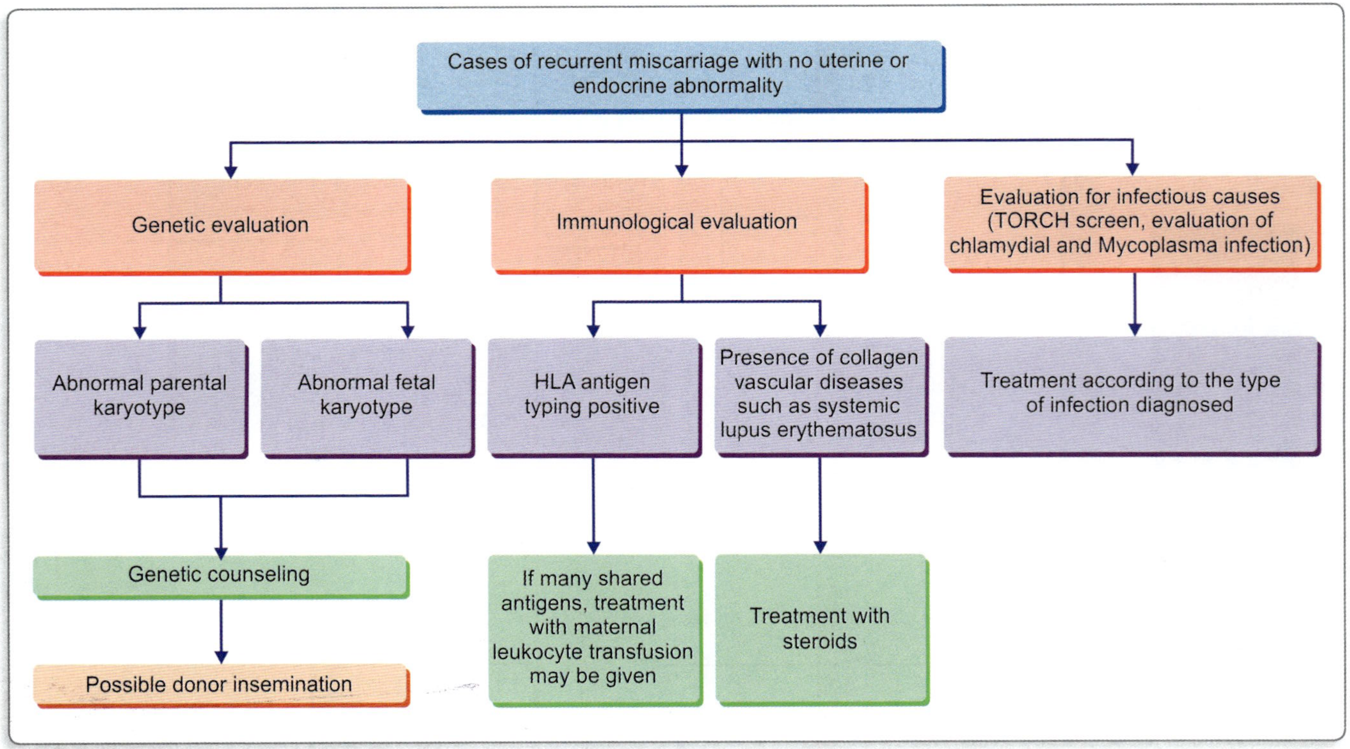

Section 3 ❖ Pregnancy-Related Complications

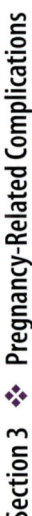

Flow Chart 15.3 Evaluation of recurrent miscarriage in cases with no endocrine or uterine anomaly on initial evaluation

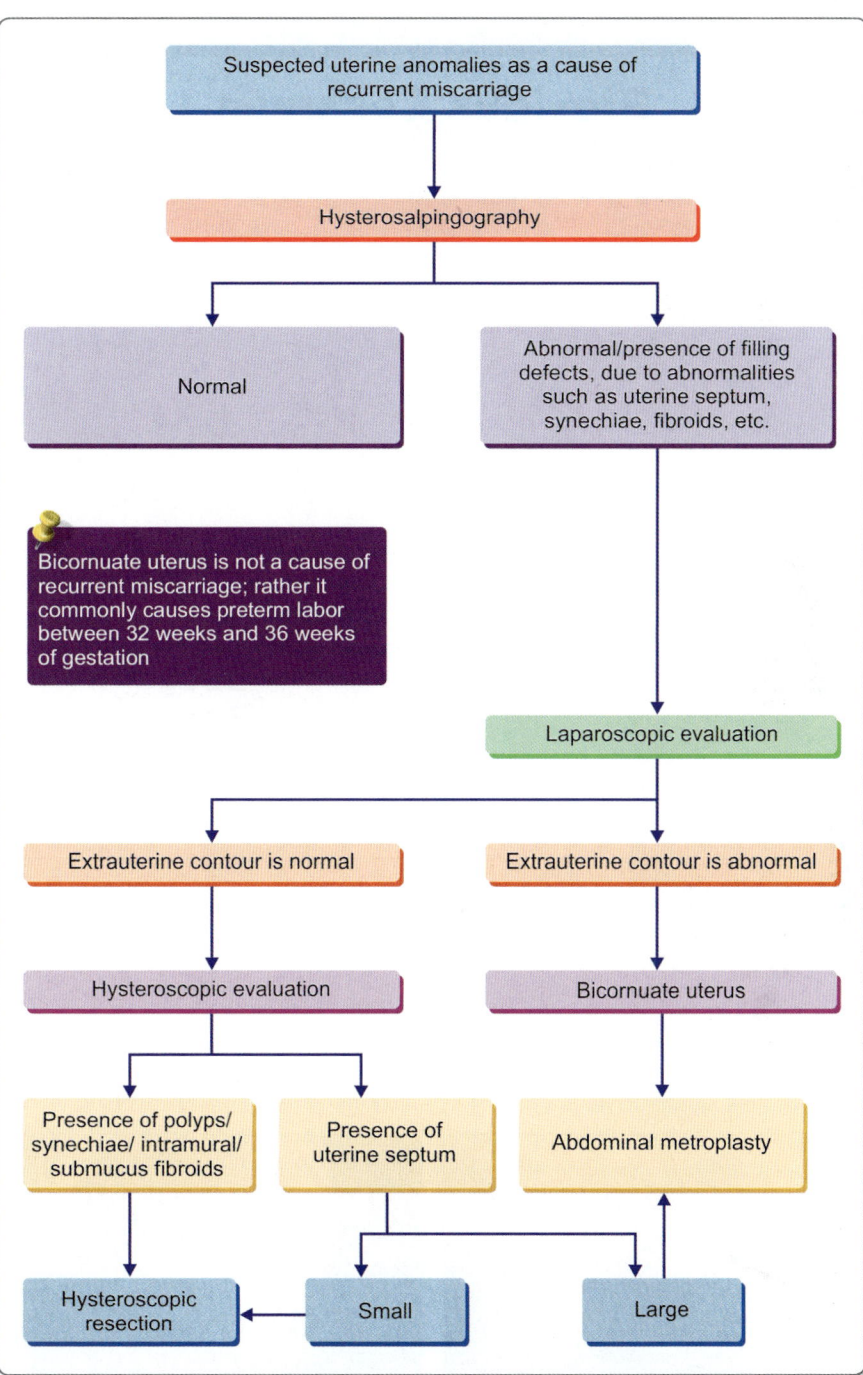

Flow Chart 15.4 Evaluation of uterine anomalies in cases of recurrent miscarriage

16 Previous Cesarean Section

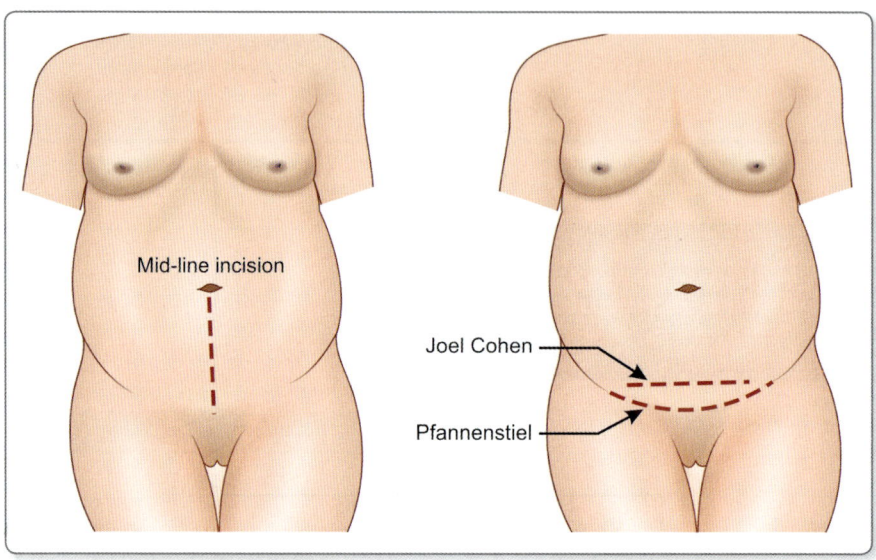

Types of abdominal skin incisions, which can be given at the time of cesarean section

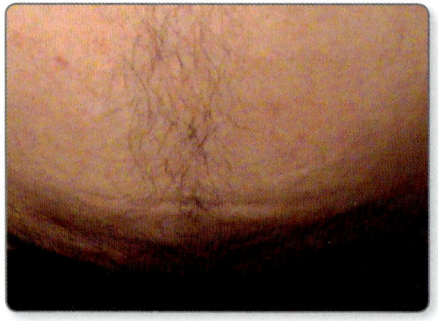

Scar mark of a previous transverse abdominal skin incision for a lower segment cesarean section

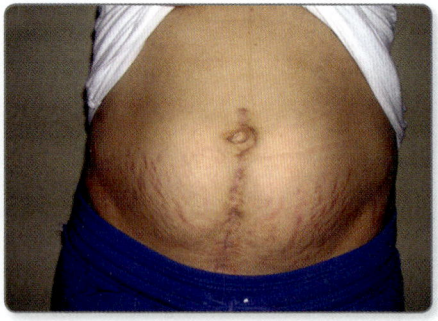

Scar mark of a previous longitudinal skin incision given at the time of cesarean delivery

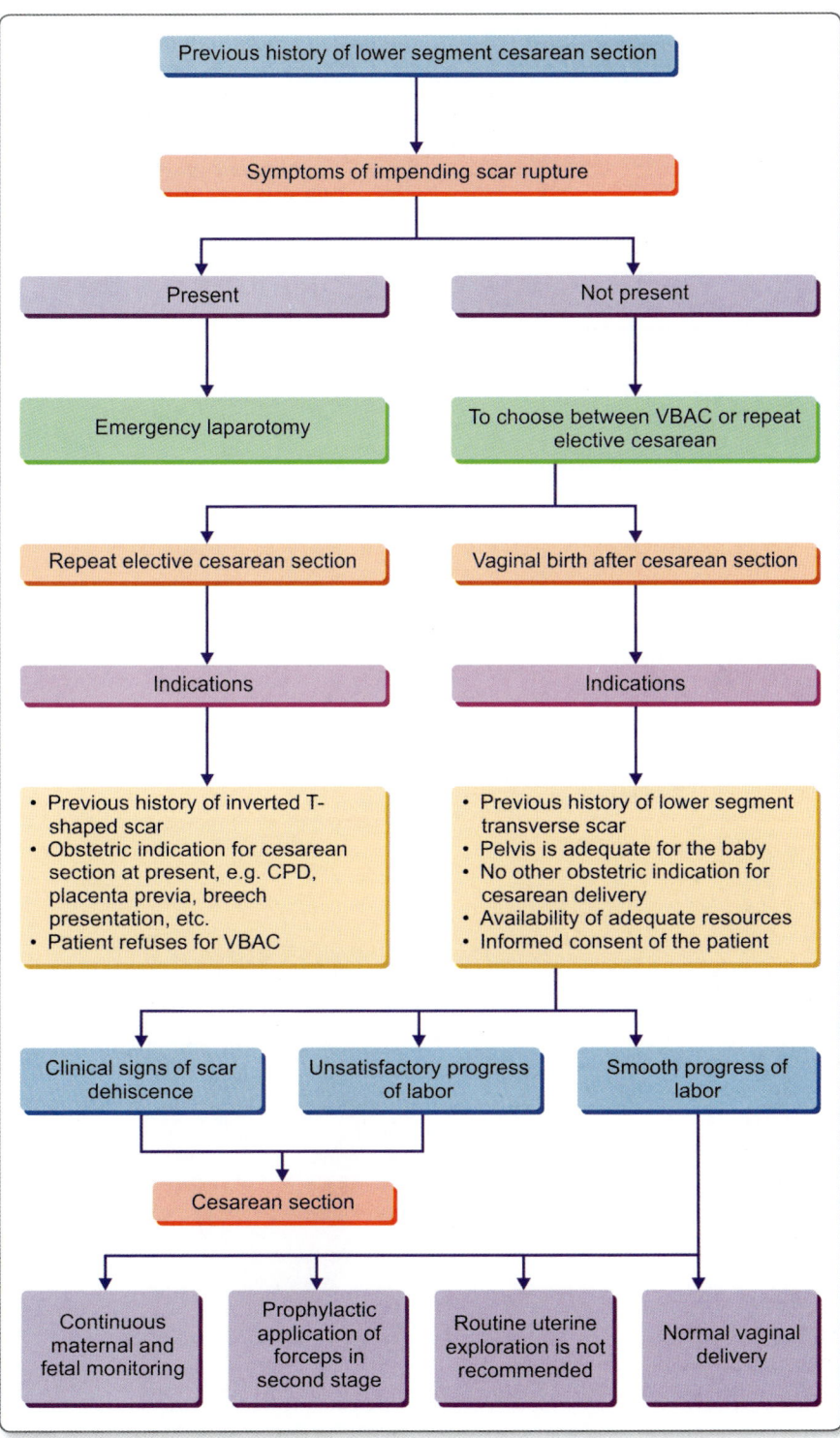

Flow Chart 16.1 Management plan of a patient with the previous history of lower segment cesarean delivery

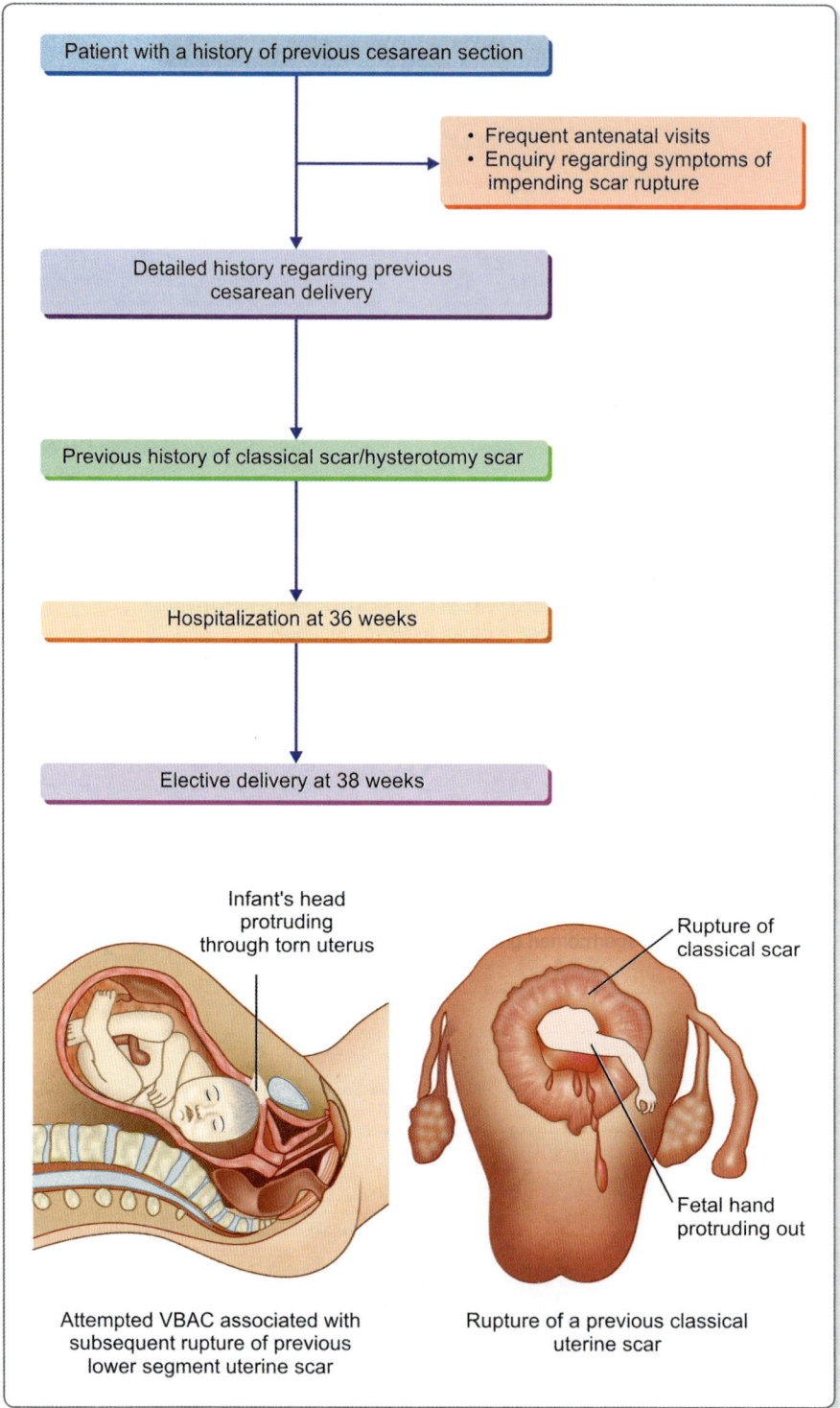

Flow Chart 16.2 Management plan of a patient with the previous history of upper segment cesarean delivery

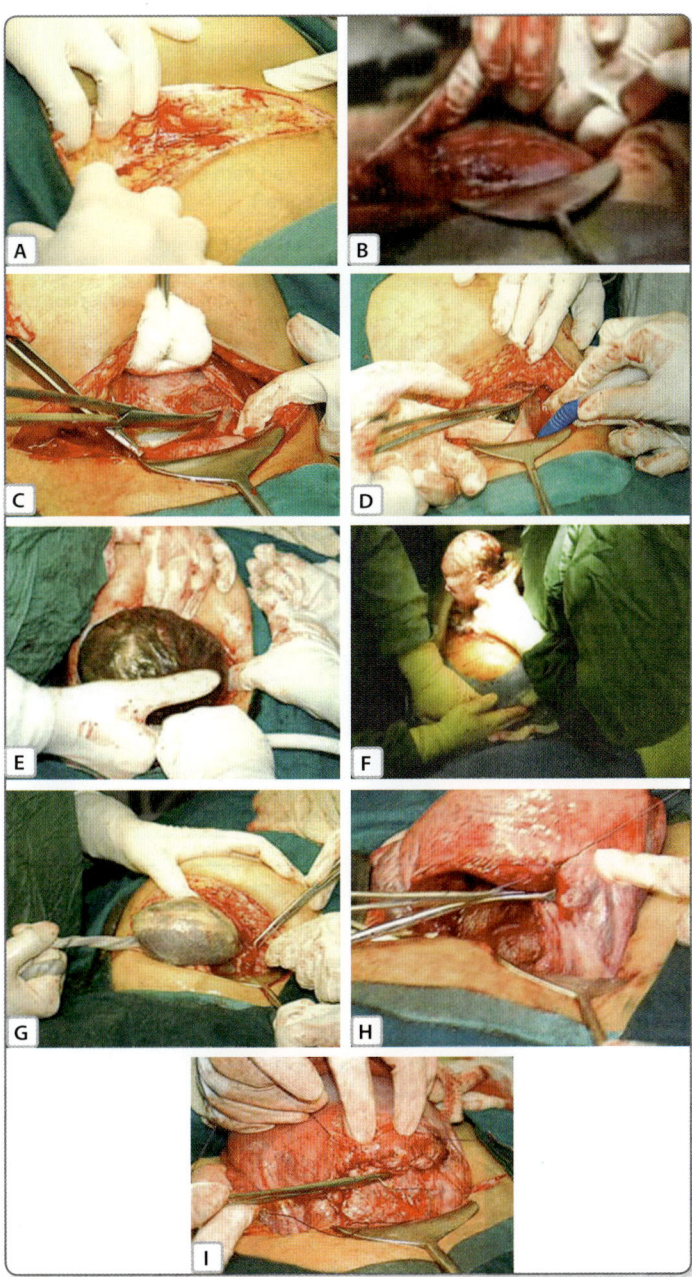

Steps of lower segment cesarean section performed using a pfannenstiel skin incision
(A) Giving an incision over the abdomen and dissecting out different layers of skin; (B) Application of Doyen's retractor after dissection of parietal peritoneum; (C) Incision of visceral peritoneum; (D) Giving a uterine incision; (E) Delivery of fetal head; (F) Delivery of the entire baby out of the uterine cavity; (G) Delivery of the placenta; (H) Clamping the uterine angles with green armytage clamps; (I) Stitching the uterine cavity

OBSTETRICS

Section 4
Medical Complications During Pregnancy

- **Chapter 17** — Preeclampsia
- **Chapter 18** — Gestational Diabetes
- **Chapter 19** — Anemia in Pregnancy
- **Chapter 20** — Heart Disease During Pregnancy
- **Chapter 21** — Asthma During Pregnancy
- **Chapter 22** — Thyroid Disorders During Pregnancy
- **Chapter 23** — Malaria in Pregnancy
- **Chapter 24** — Pregnancy in Obese Women

17 Preeclampsia

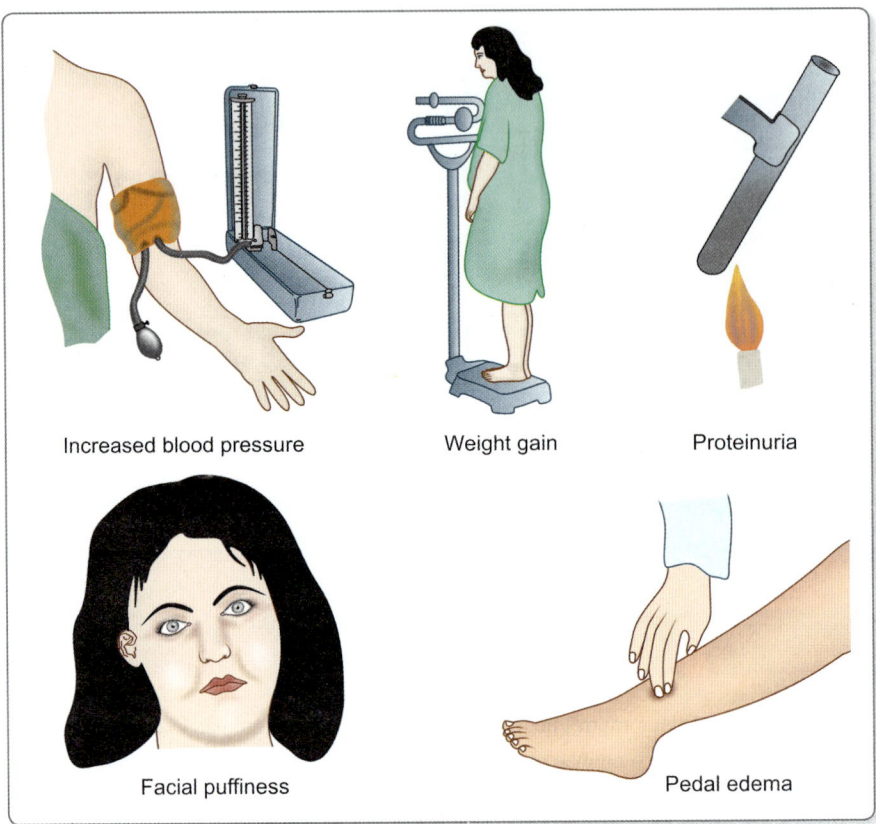

Clinical features of preeclampsia

Definition
Preeclampsia can be defined as the presence of high blood pressure and proteinuria, which develop after the 20th week of pregnancy and goes away after the delivery.

Characteristics of preeclampsia
- Appearance of high BP (> 140/90 mm Hg) for the first time during pregnancy after 20 weeks of gestation
- Presence of proteinuria (> 300 mg/L or > 1 + on the dipstick)
- BP returns to normal within 12 weeks of postpartum period

Definition and characteristics of preeclampsia

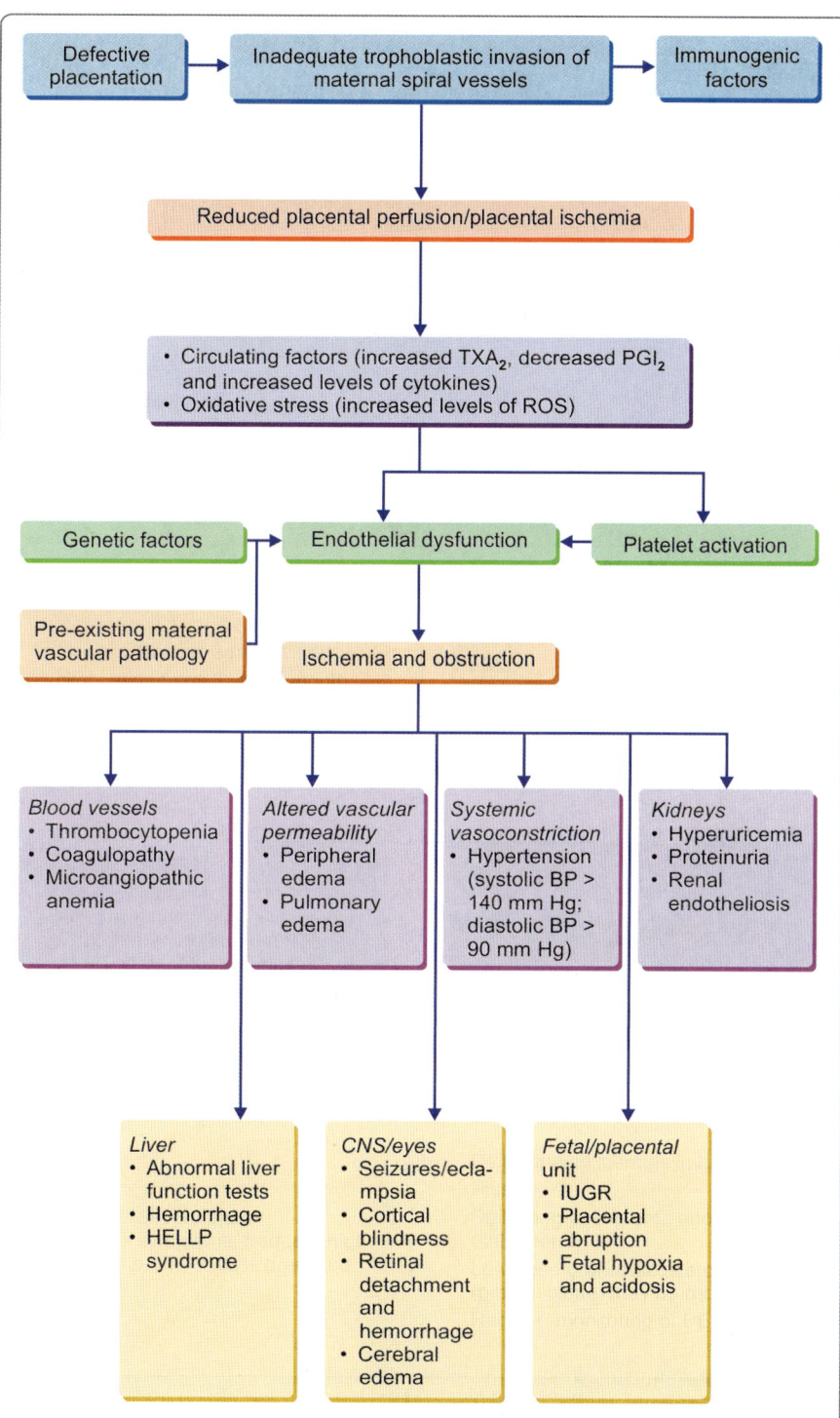

Flow Chart 17.1 Pathophysiology of preeclampsia

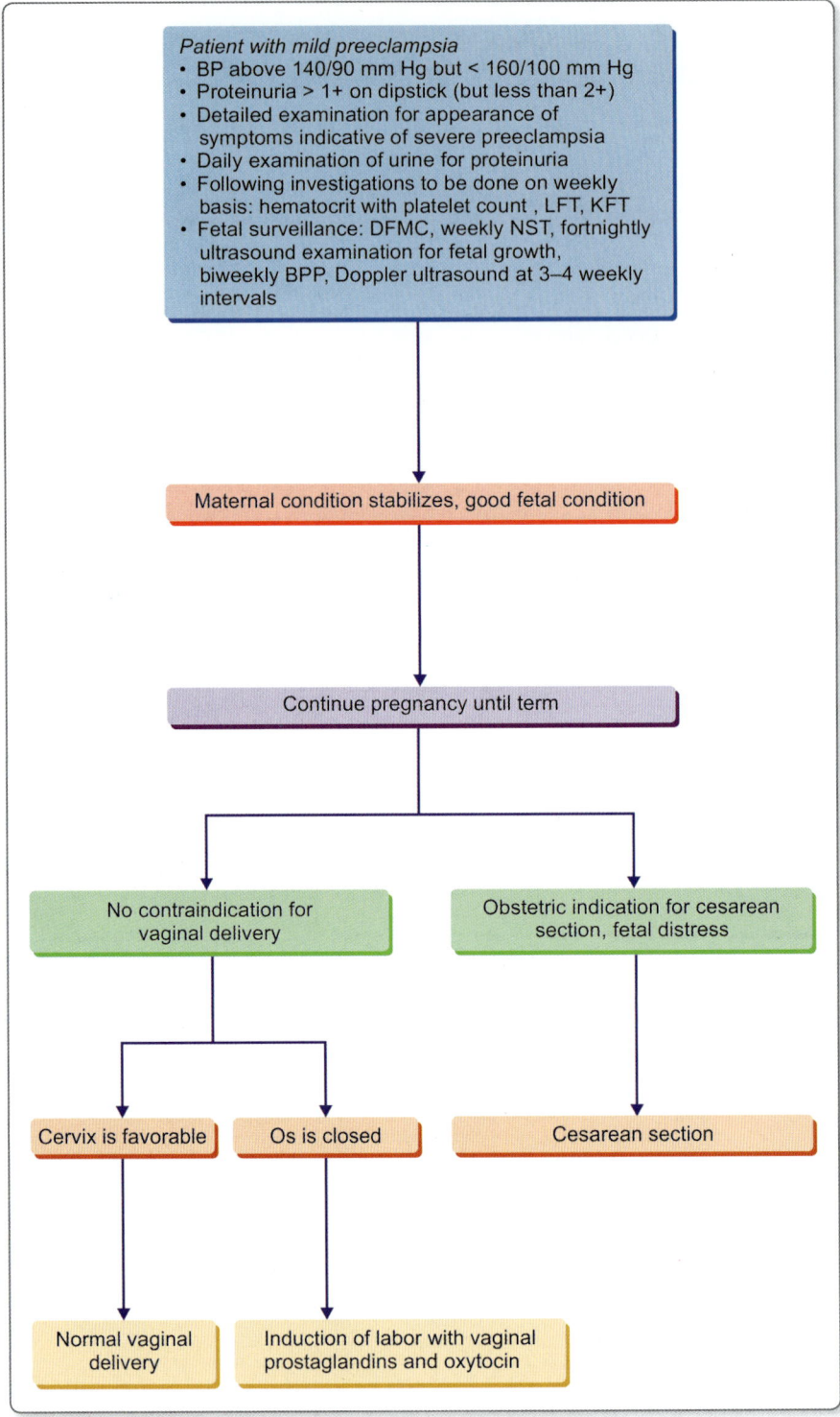

Flow Chart 17.2 Management of cases of mild preeclampsia

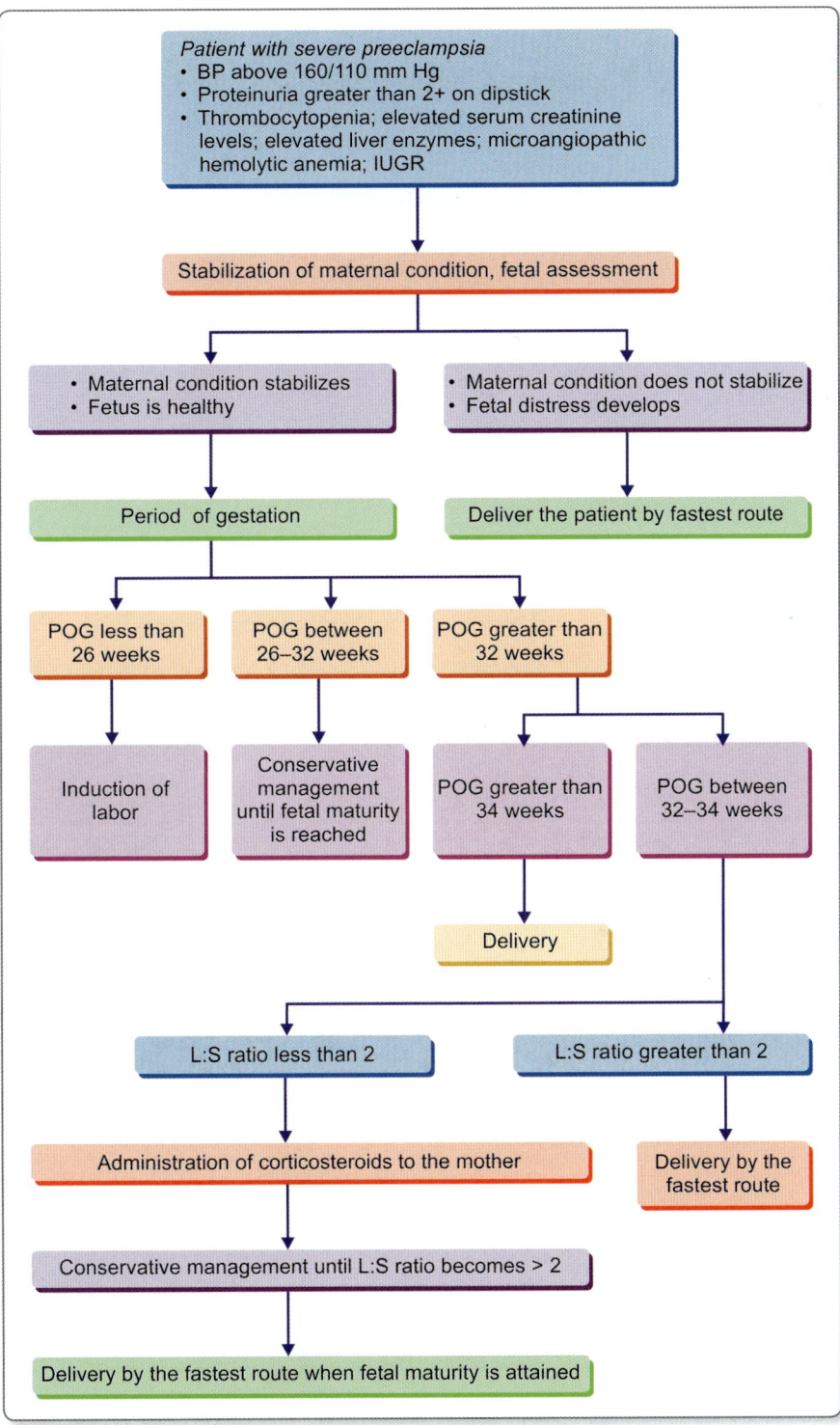

Flow Chart 17.3 Management of cases with severe preeclampsia

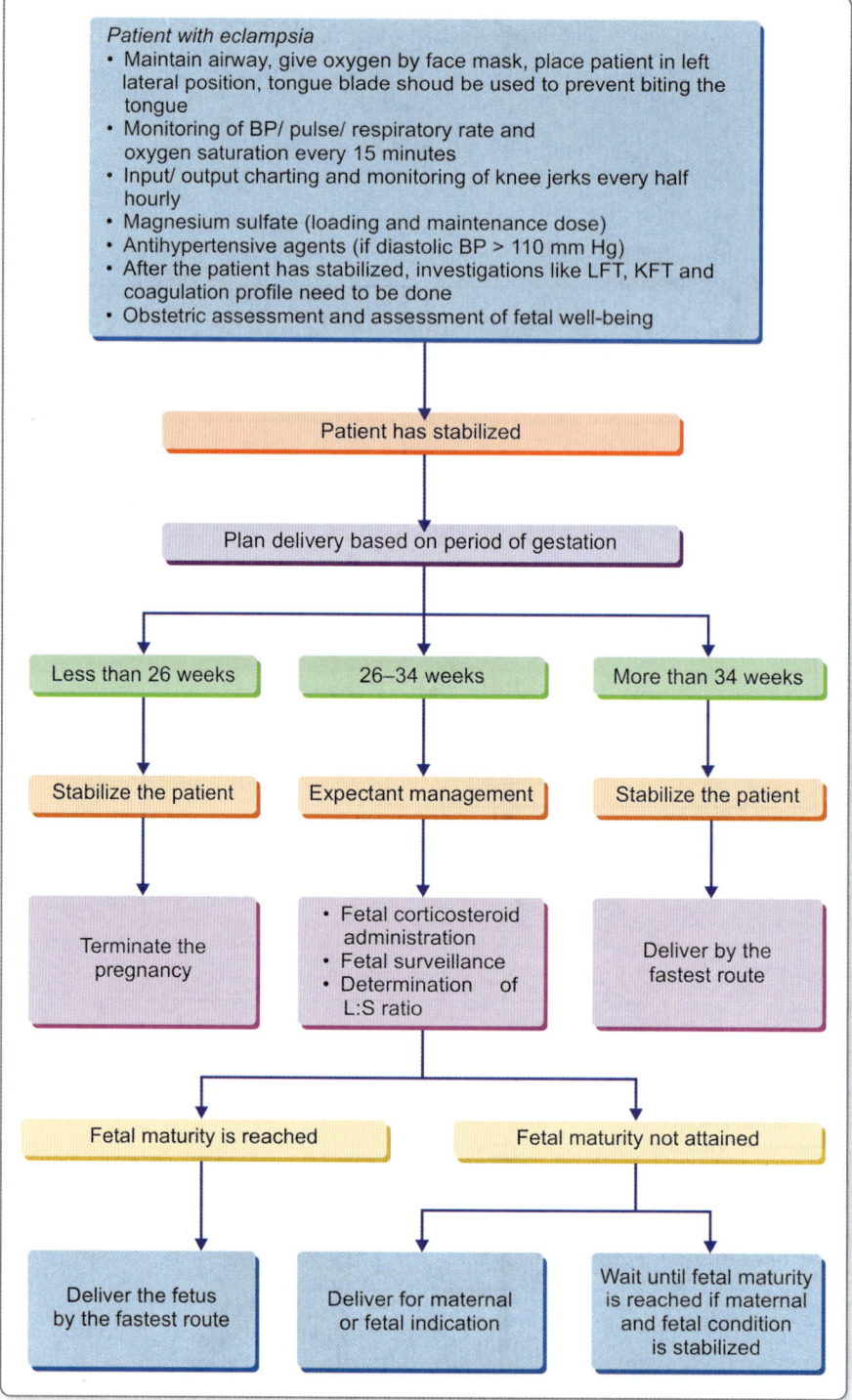

Flow Chart 17.4　Management of cases with eclampsia

18. Gestational Diabetes

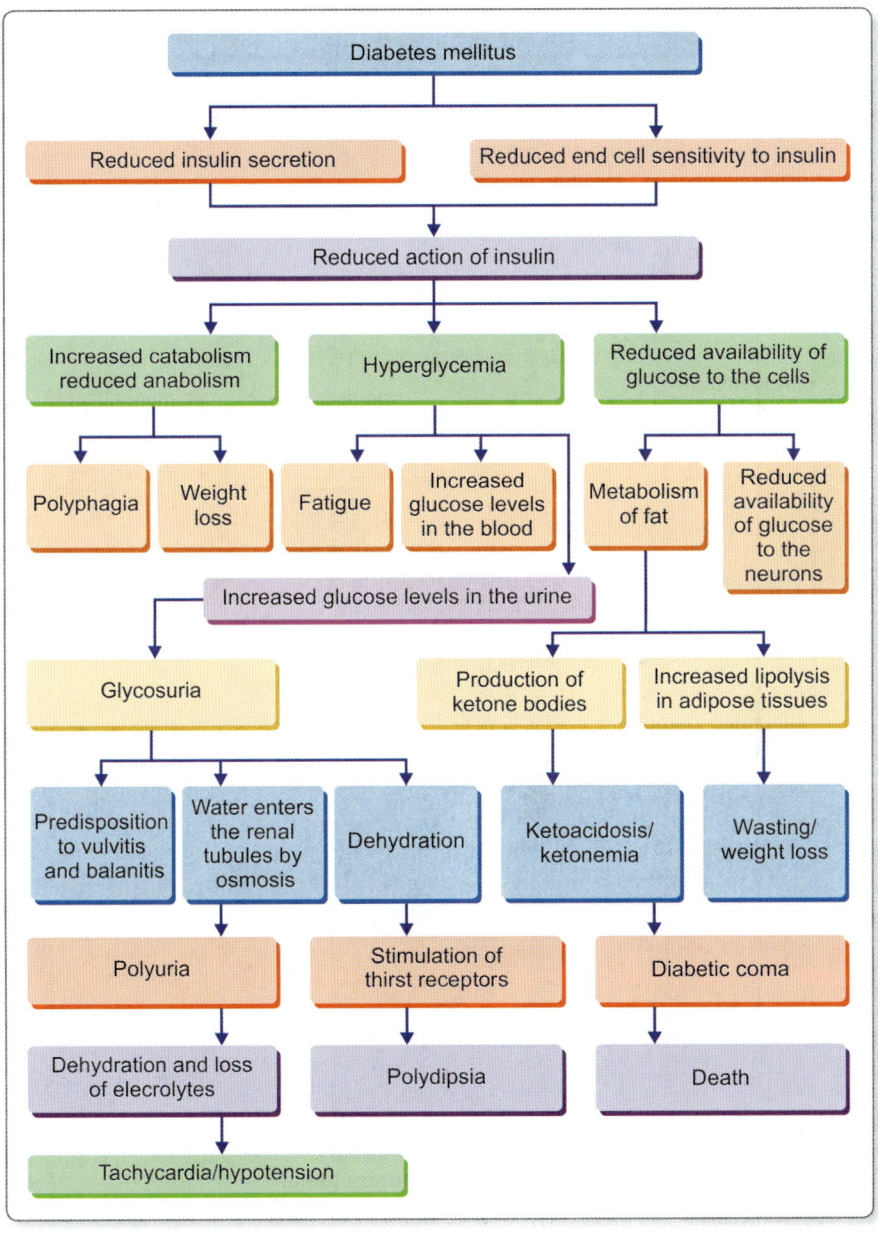

Flow Chart 18.1 Immediate metabolic consequences of diabetes mellitus

Section 4 ❖ Medical Complications During Pregnancy

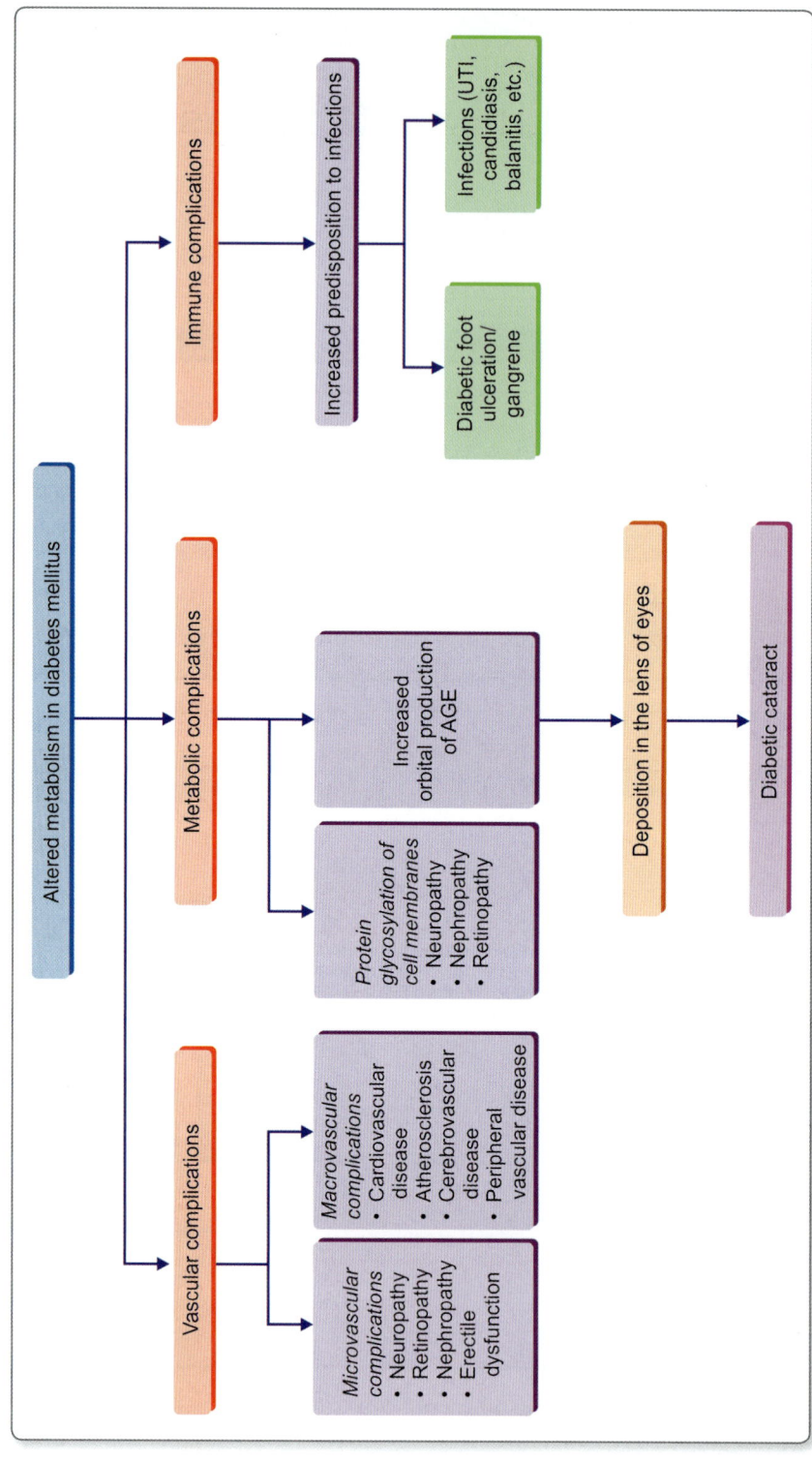

Flow Chart 18.2 Delayed complications of diabetes mellitus

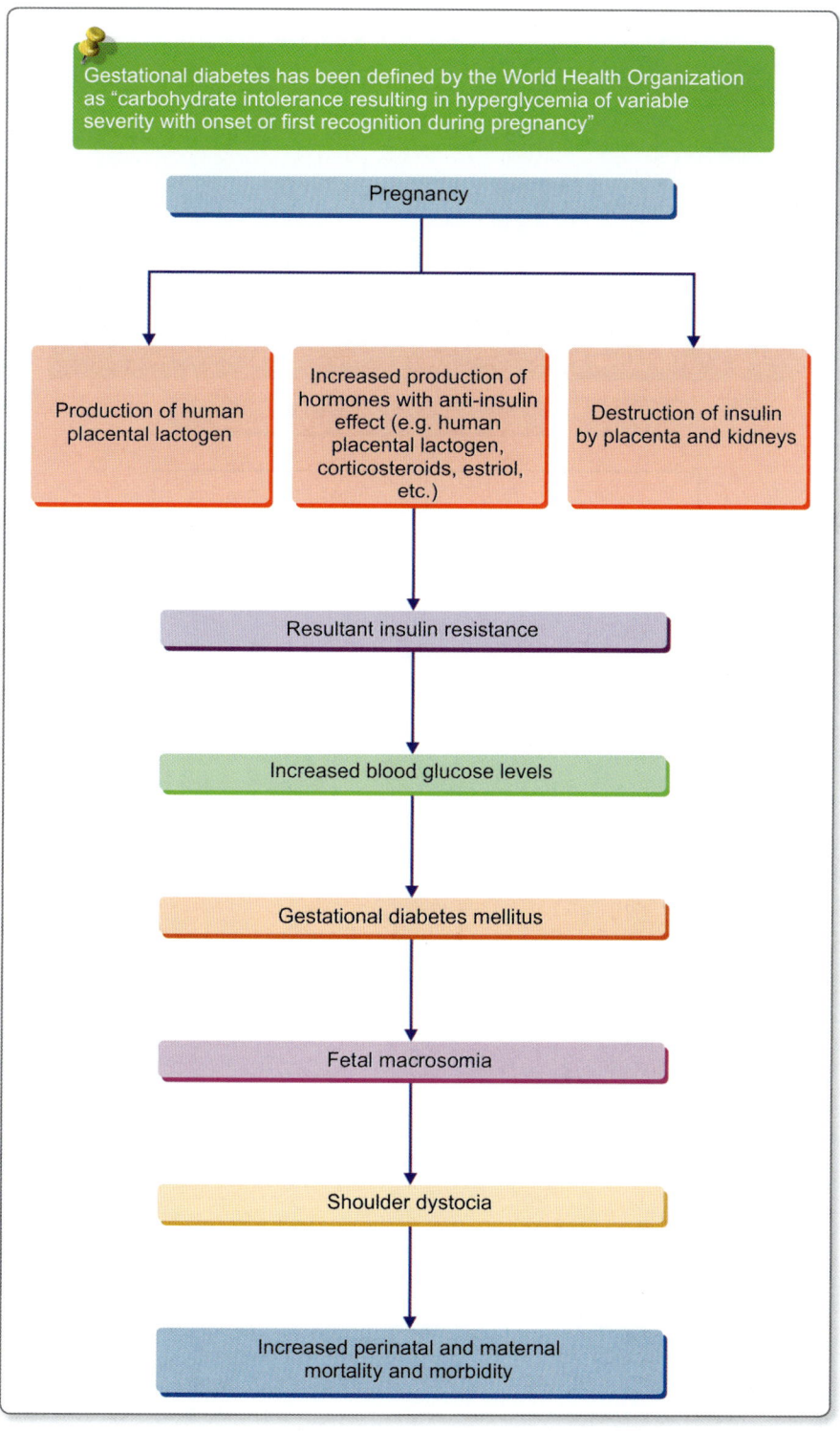

Flow Chart 18.3 Pathogenesis of gestational diabetes

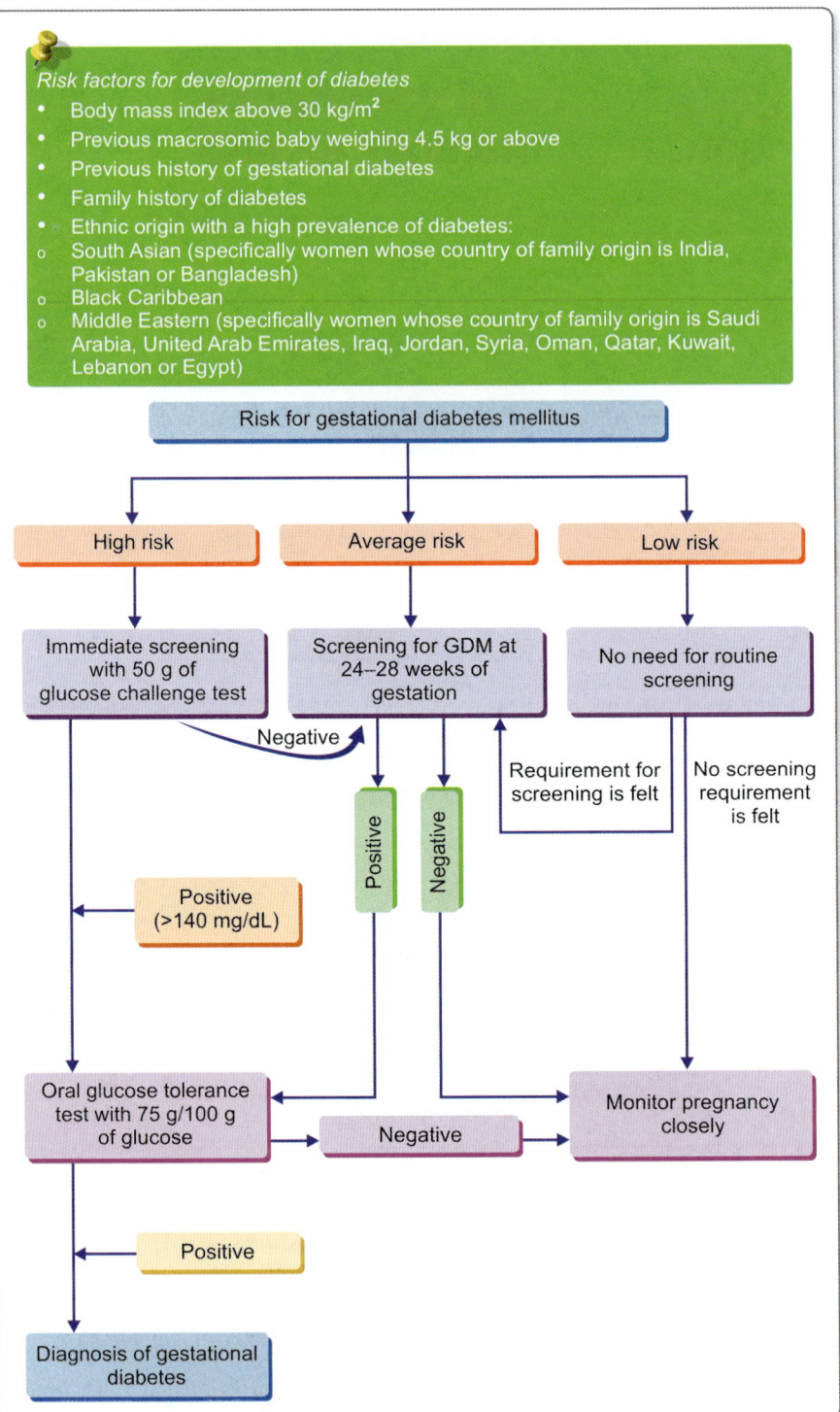

Flow Chart 18.4 Screening for gestational diabetes

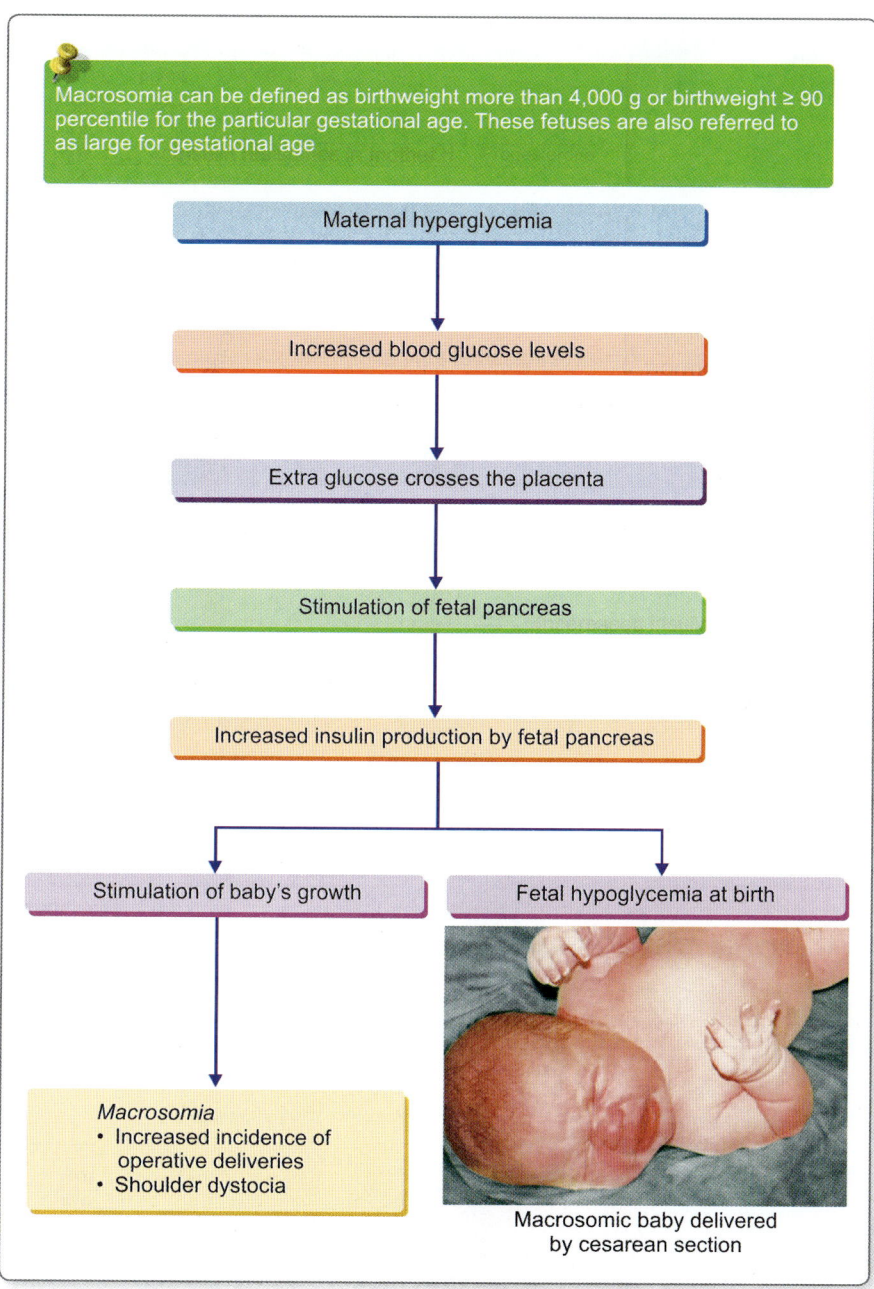

Flow Chart 18.5 Pathogenesis of fetal macrosomia

19 Anemia in Pregnancy

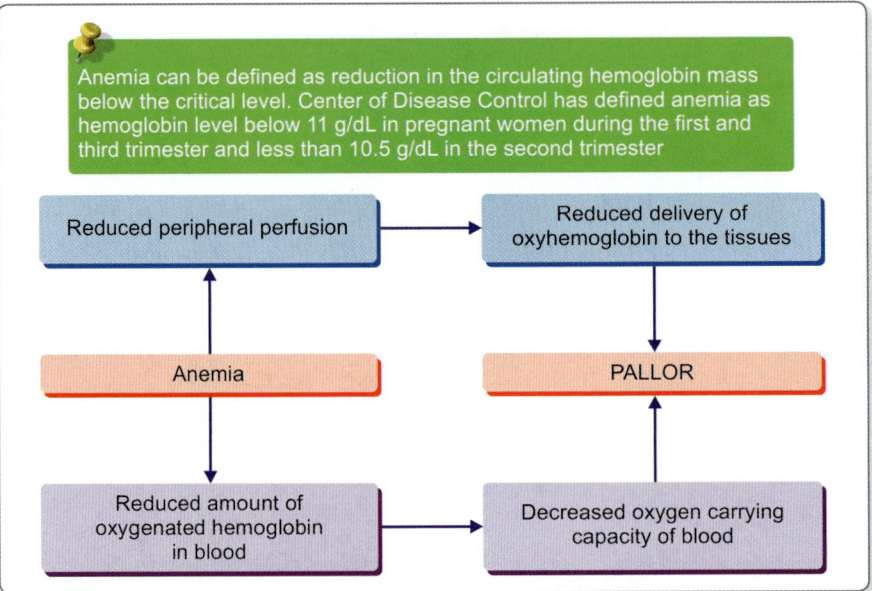

Flow Chart 19.1 Mechanism of development of pallor in anemic patients

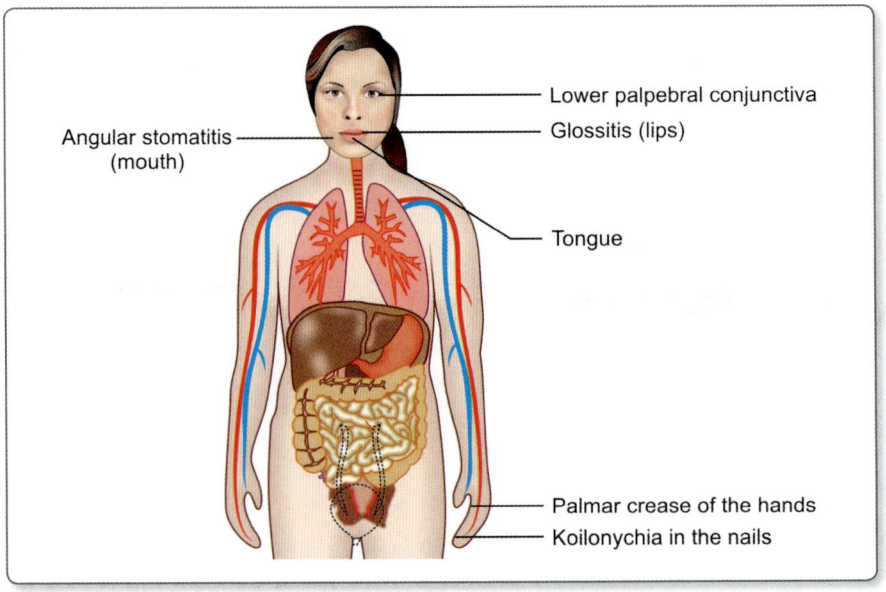

Areas to look for pallor in the human body

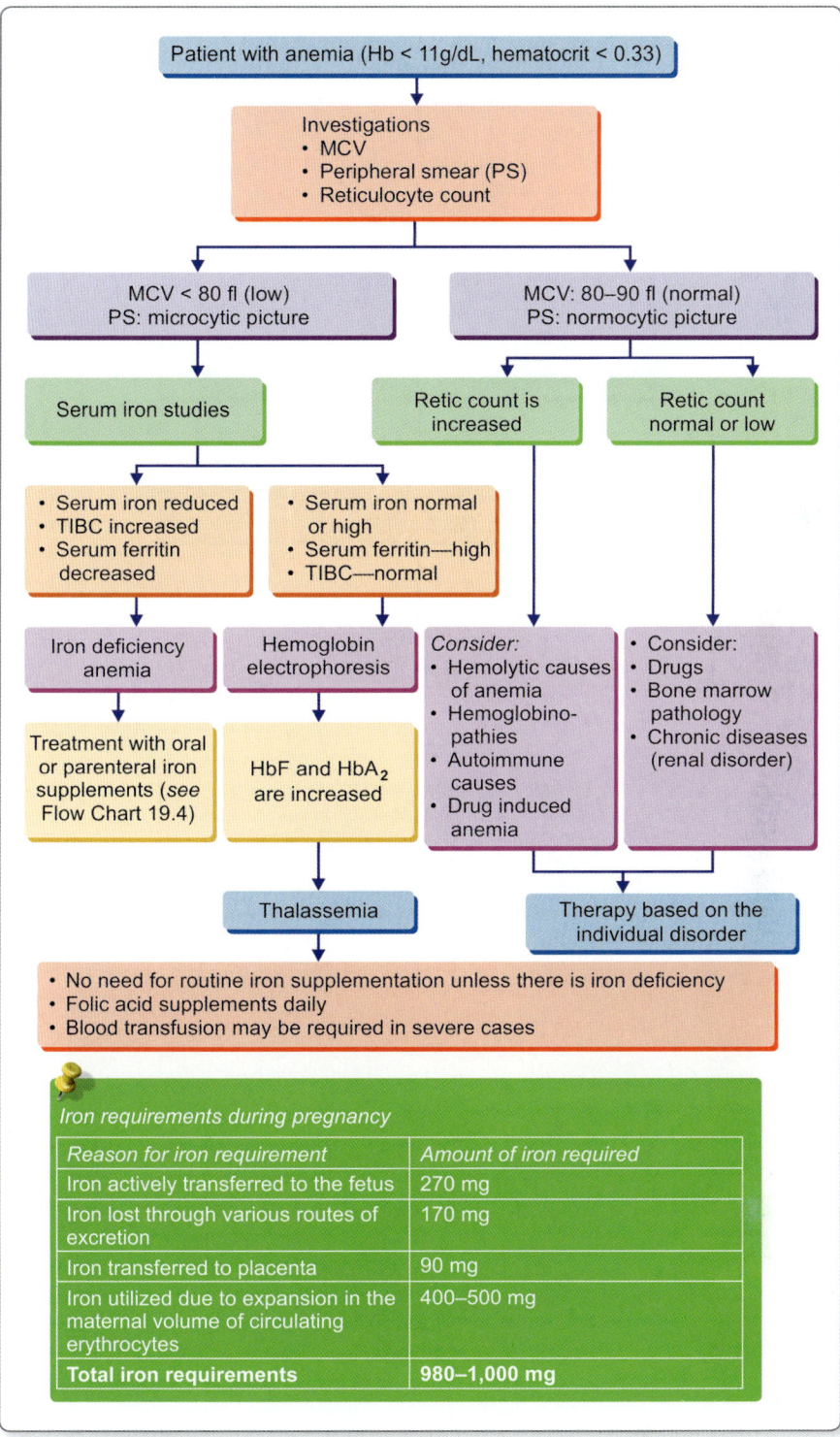

Flow Chart 19.2 Diagnosis of microcytic and normocytic anemia during pregnancy

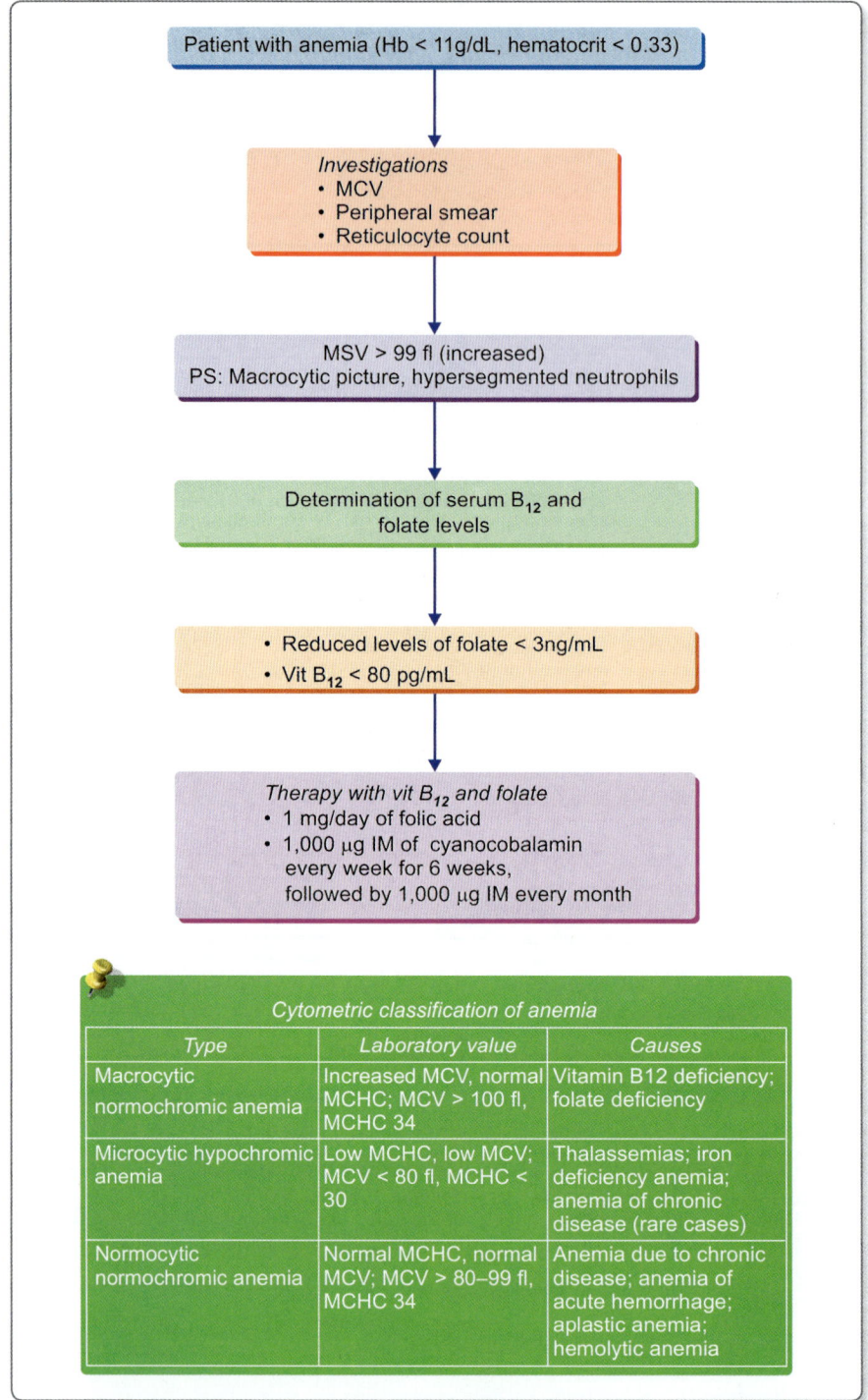

Flow Chart 19.3 Diagnosis of macrocytic anemia during pregnancy

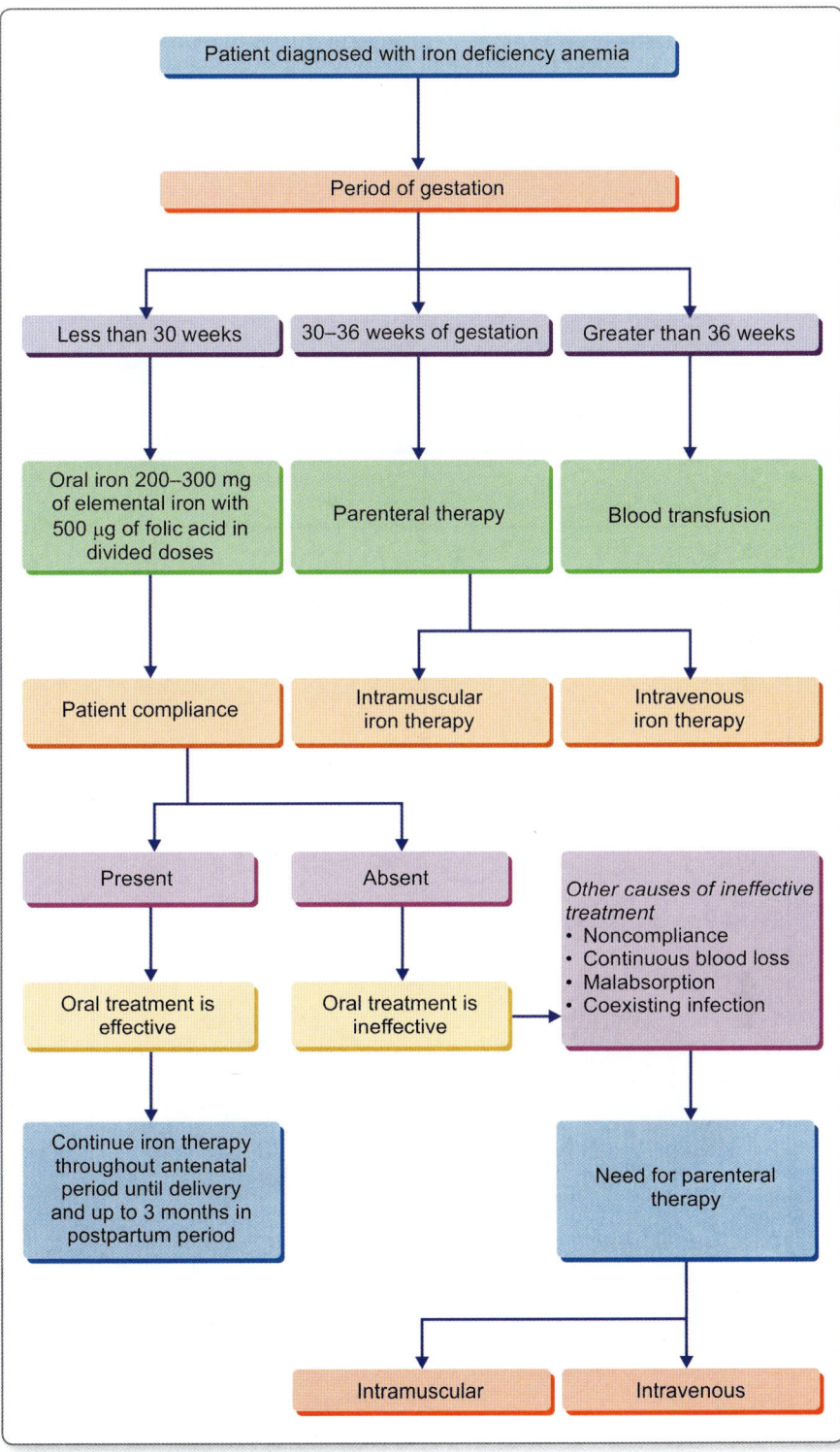

Flow Chart 19.4 Treatment of iron deficiency anemia in pregnancy

20. Heart Disease During Pregnancy

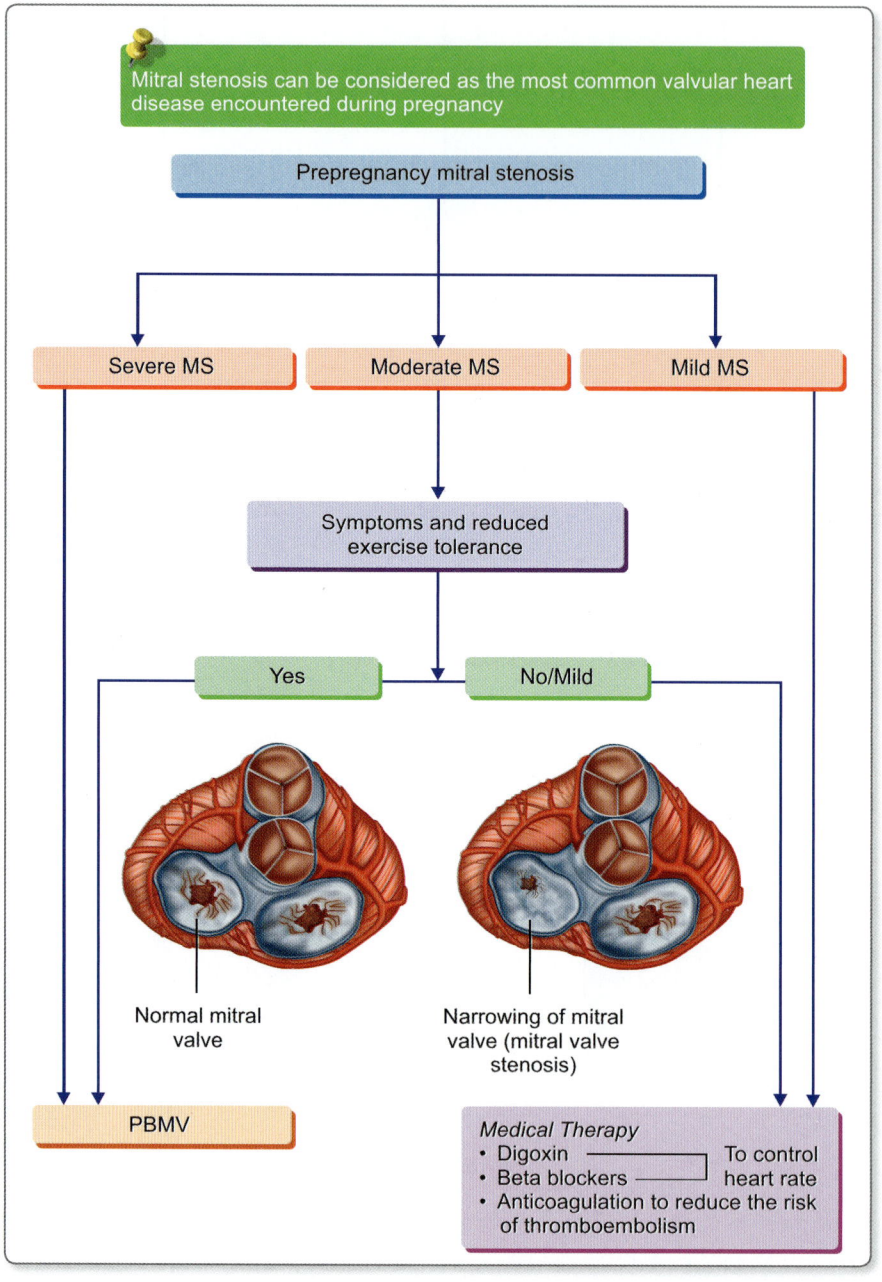

Flow Chart 20.1 Management of women with mitral stenosis diagnosed prior to pregnancy

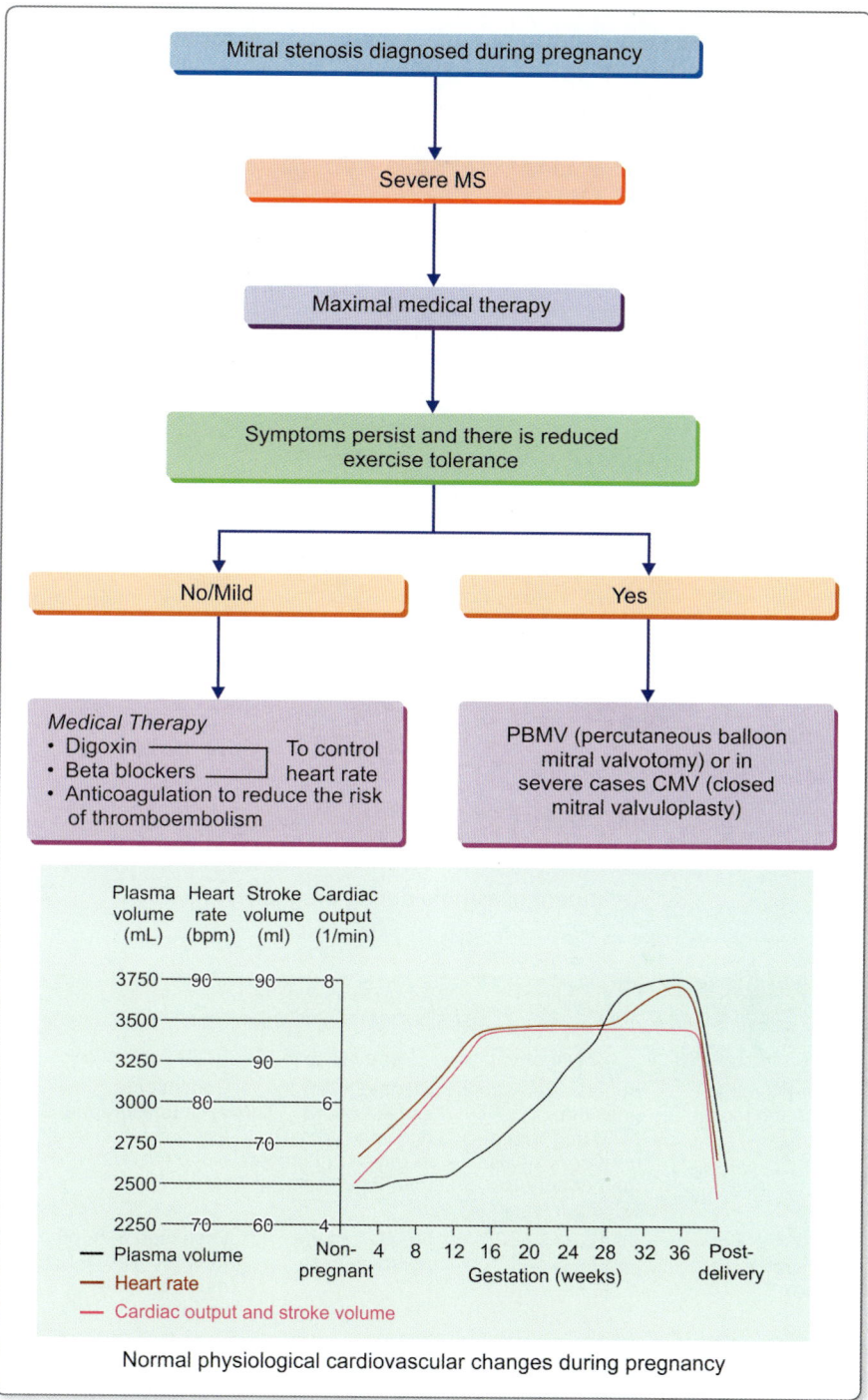

Flow Chart 20.2 Management of women with mitral stenosis diagnosed during pregnancy

21 Asthma During Pregnancy

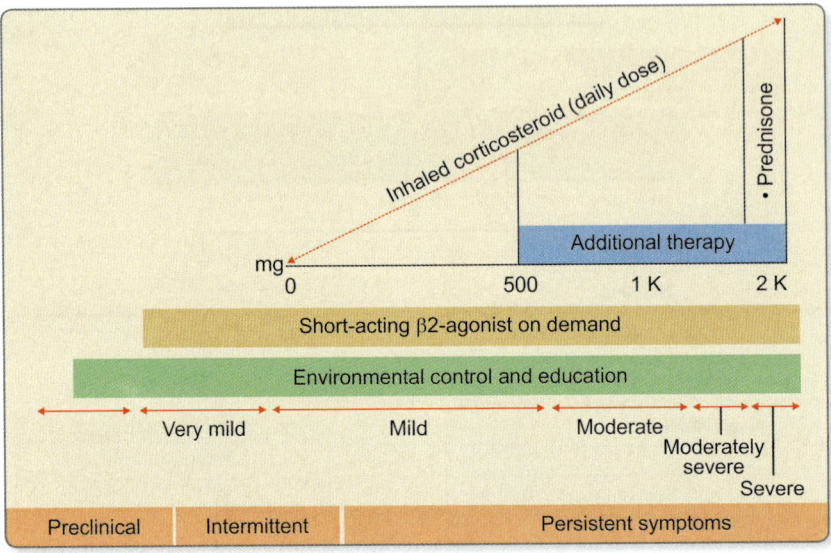

Treatment of asthma during pregnancy

Classification of asthma by National Asthma Education Program (NAEP)			
Characteristics	Mild asthma	Moderate asthma	Severe asthma
Symptomatic exacerbations	Brief exacerbations (less than 1 hour) occurring with a frequency of less than or equal to twice per week	Symptomatic exacerbations occurring with a frequency of greater than 2 per week	Continuous symptoms/frequent exacerbations limit activity levels
PEFR (Peak expiratory flow rate)	≥ 80% of the personal best	60–80% of the personal best	Less than 60% of the predicted and may be highly variable
FEV1	≥ 80% of the predicted when asymptomatic	60–80% of the predicted	Less than 60% of the predicted and may be highly variable
Nocturnal symptoms	None	Nocturnal symptoms may be present	Nocturnal symptoms are present

Asthma as classified by NAEP

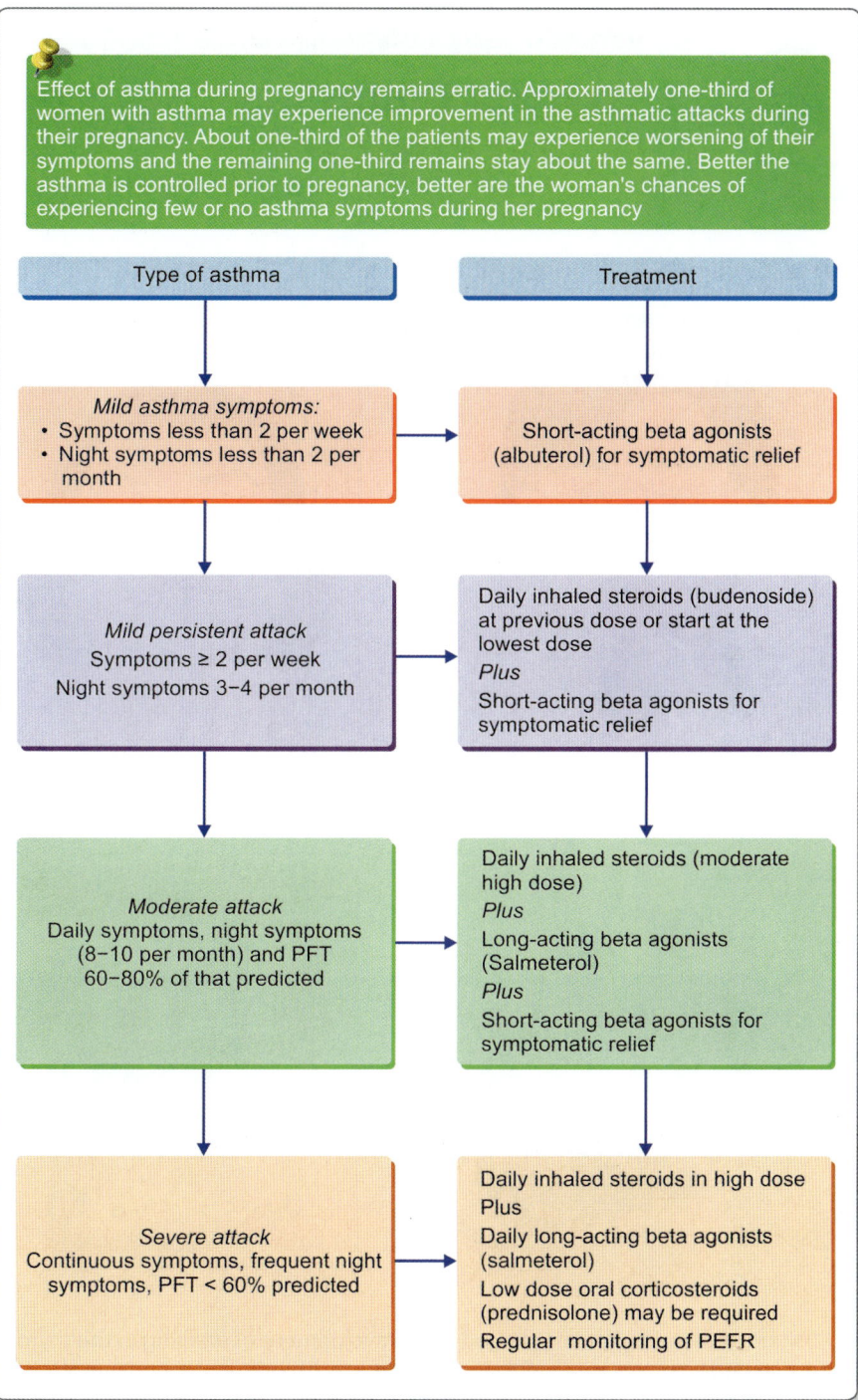

Flow Chart 21.1 Management of asthma based on the severity of symptoms during pregnancy

22 Thyroid Disorders During Pregnancy

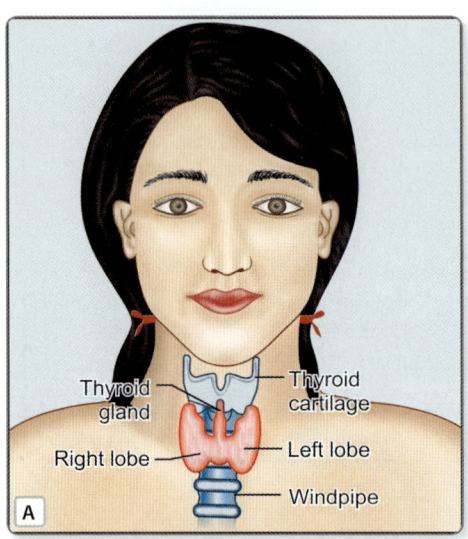
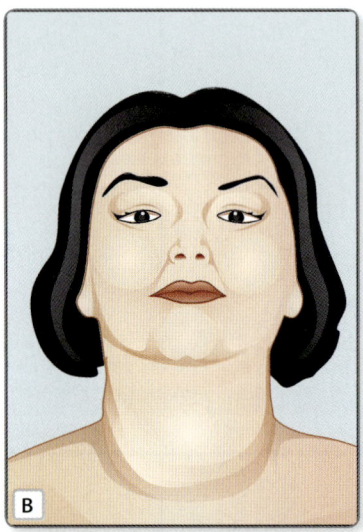
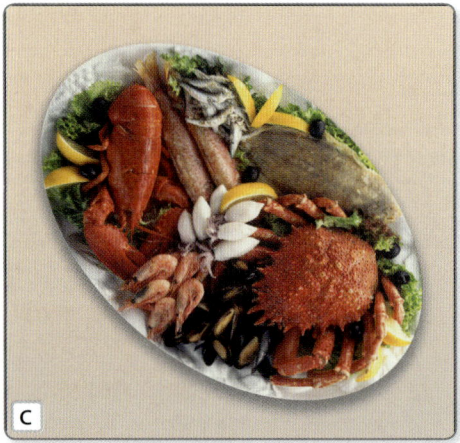
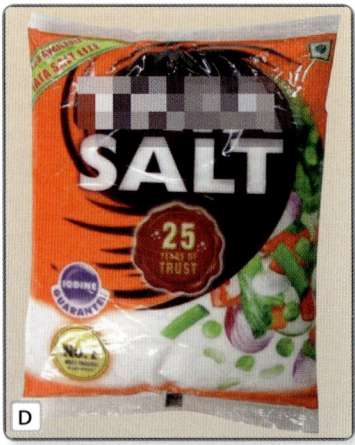

(A) Position of thyroid gland in the body; (B) Development of swelling in the thyroid gland known as goiter; (C) Seafood: a rich source of iodine; (D) Consumption of iodized salt helps in preventing iodine deficiency

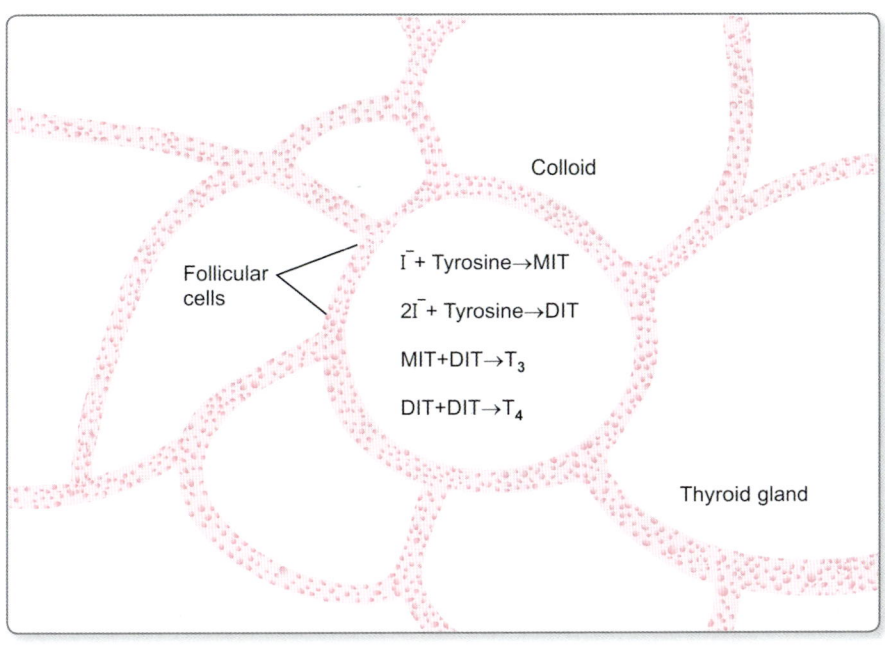

Flow Chart 22.1 Synthesis of thyroid hormones

Changes in the thyroid function tests during normal pregnancy	
Physiologic change	Resulting change in thyroid activity
Increased level of serum estrogens	Rise in the levels of thyroid hormone transport proteins (serum TBG)
Increased serum TBG	Increase in total T_4 and T_3
Increase in hCG levels	Stimulates the production of T_3 and T_4 from the thyroid gland Reciprocal decrease in serum TSH concentration
Increased iodine clearance	Increased dietary requirement for I^- (reduced hormone production in I^- deficient areas results in development of goiter)
Increased production of type III deiodinase by placenta	Increased T_4 and T_3 degradation Increased demand for T_4 and T_3 Compensatory increase in thyroid volume

Thyroid function tests during normal pregnancy

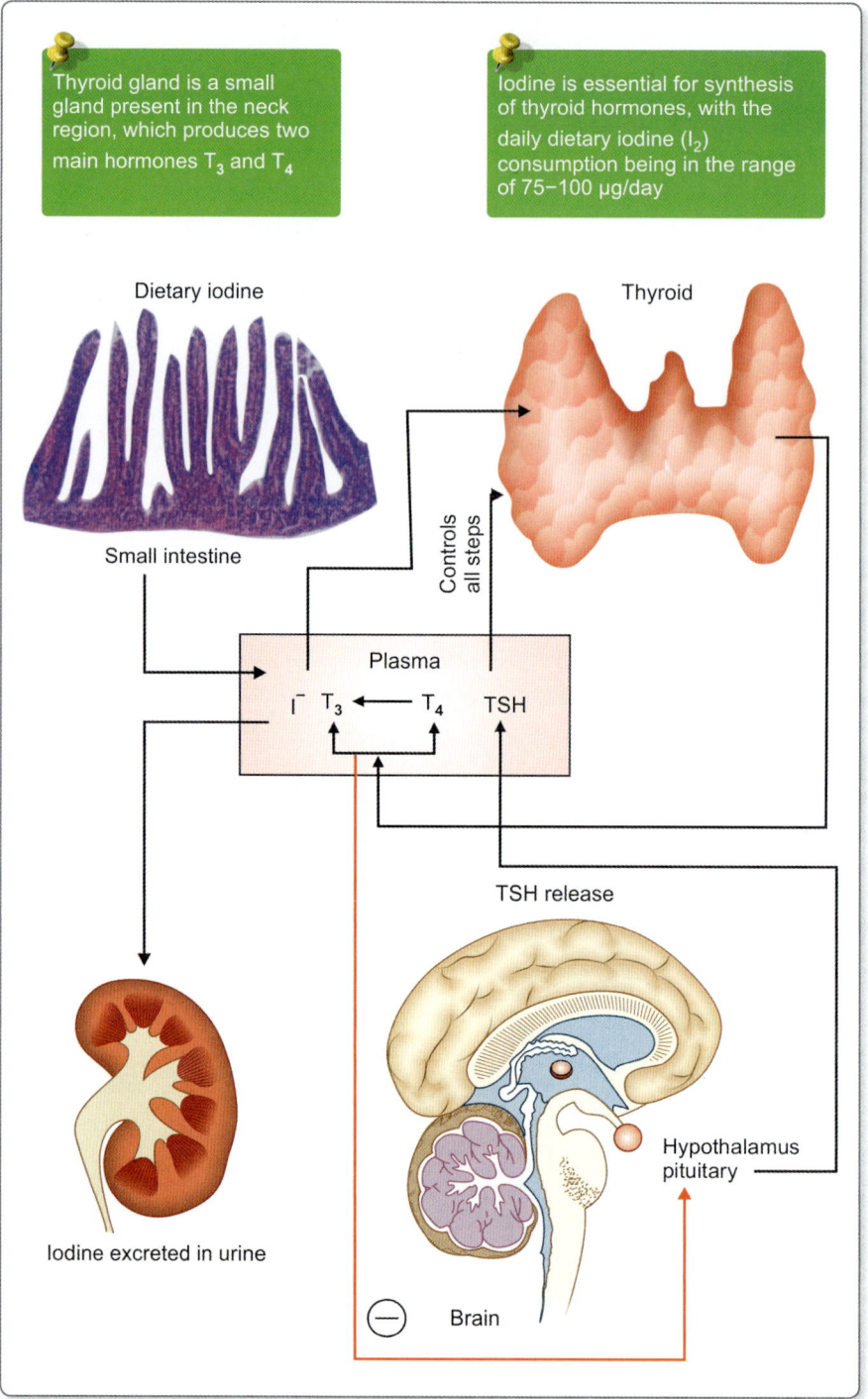

Flow Chart 22.2 Normal thyroid physiology

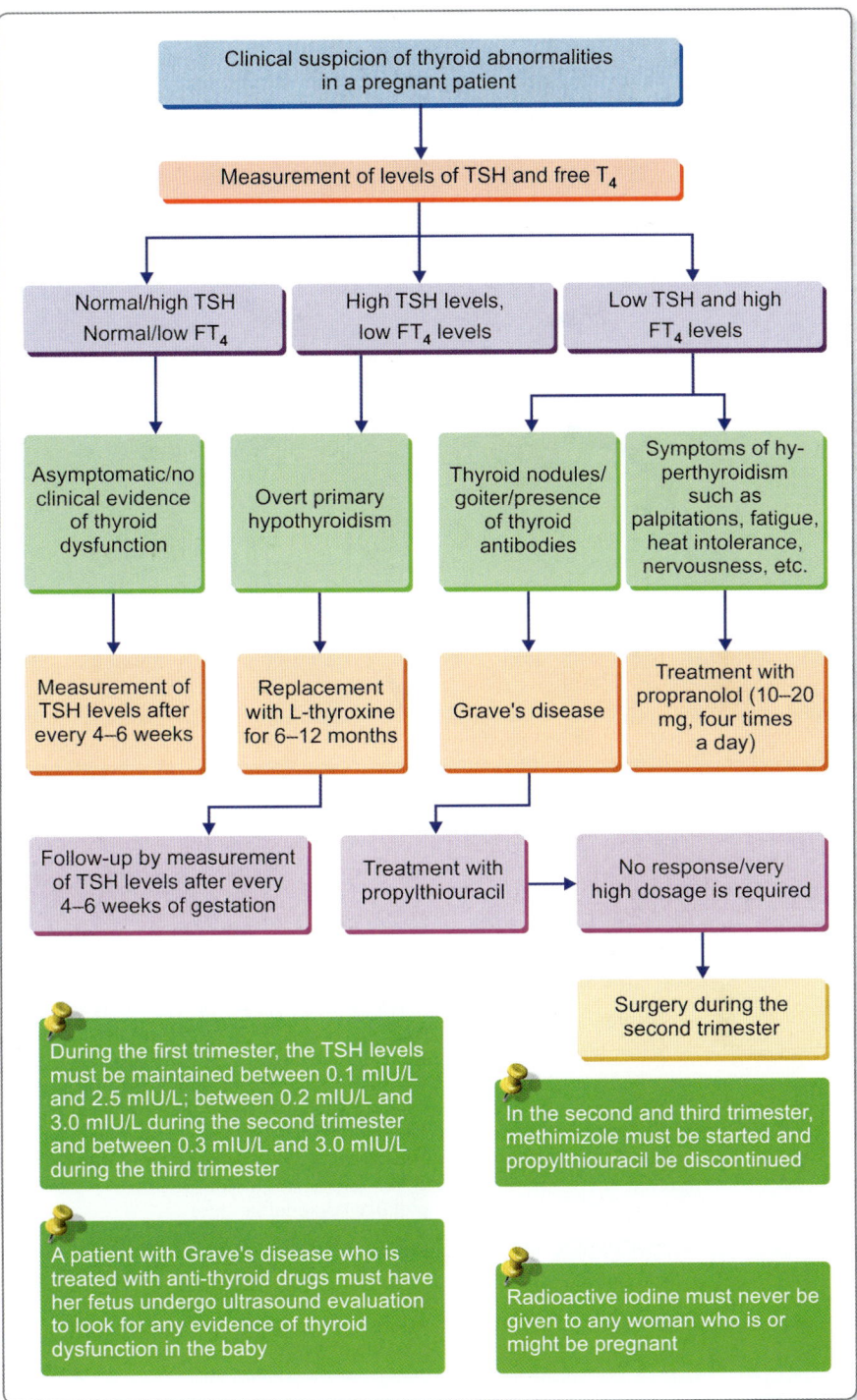

Flow Chart 22.3 Management of thyroid disorders during pregnancy

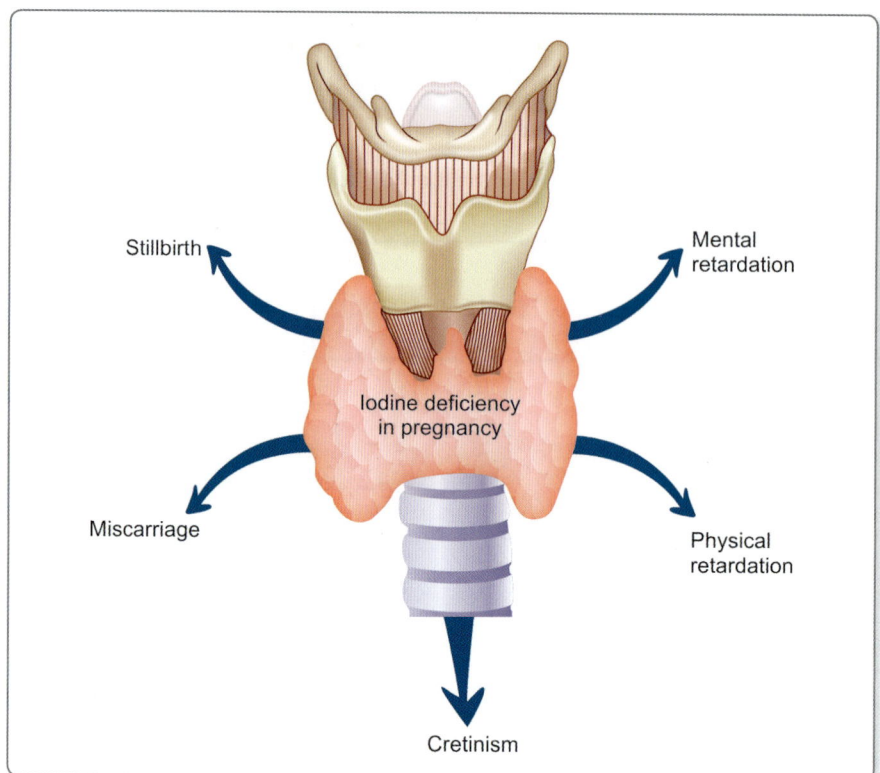

Flow Chart 22.4 Consequences of iodine deficiency during pregnancy

The spectrum of iodine deficiency disorders	
Disorder	Symptoms
Goiter	Small thyroid enlargement (grade 1) Medium thyroid enlargement (grade 2) Massive thyroid enlargement (grade 3) Multinodular goiter
Symptoms of hypothyroidism	Combination of clinical signs (hoarse voice, decreased metabolic rate, pretibial myxedema, etc.)
Physical and mental retardation	Subnormal intelligence, delayed milestones, hearing and speech defects, strabismus, nystagmus, etc.
Neurological cretinism	Severely stunted physical and mental growth, spasticity, muscular weakness in legs, arms, trunks, etc.

Iodine deficiency disorders and their symptoms

23 Malaria in Pregnancy

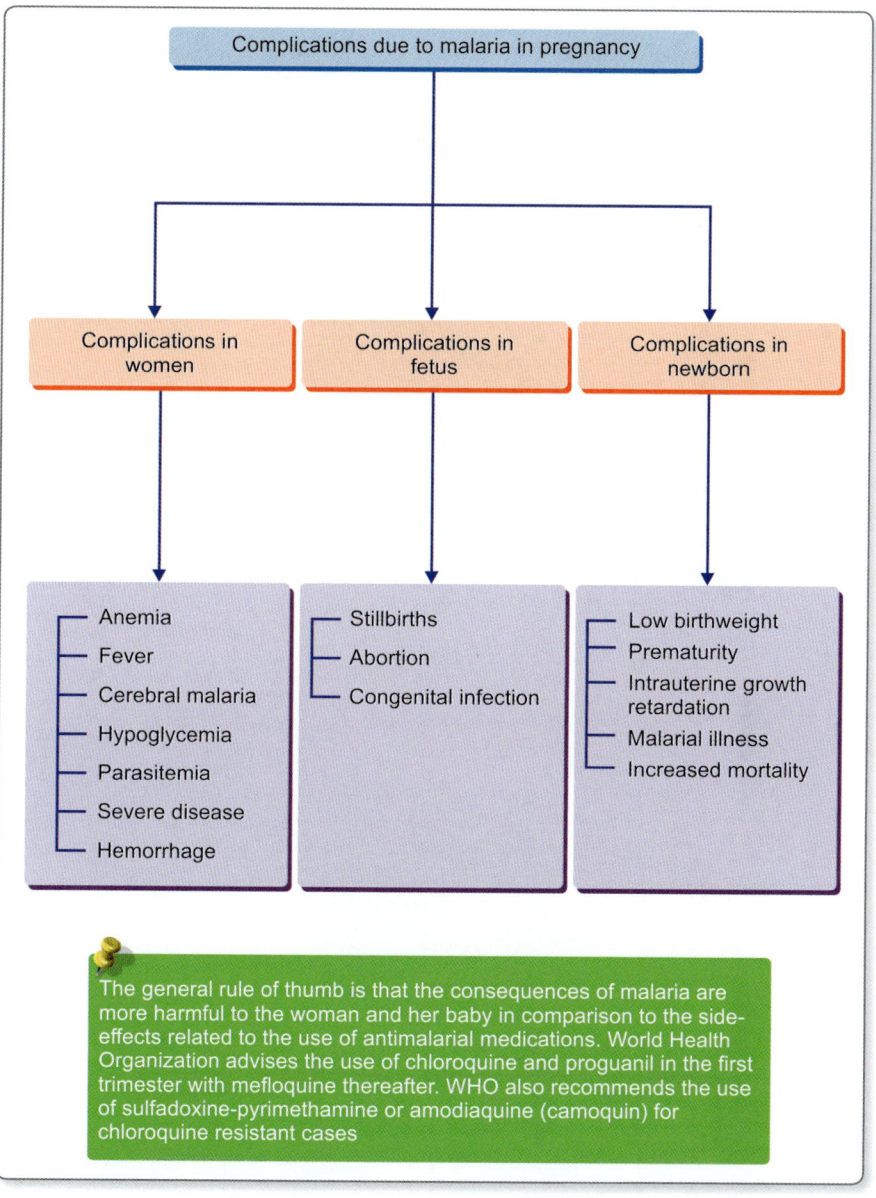

Flow Chart 23.1   Complications due to malaria in pregnancy

24. Pregnancy in Obese Women

Obesity is defined as body mass index (BMI = Wt/ht^2 = kg/m^2 × 100 = $lb/inch^2$ × 1,000) of greater than 30

Besides the adverse effects on pregnancy outcome, obesity is not only a known risk factor for subfertility due to anovulation, but it is also associated with lower pregnancy rates in subfertile ovulatory women

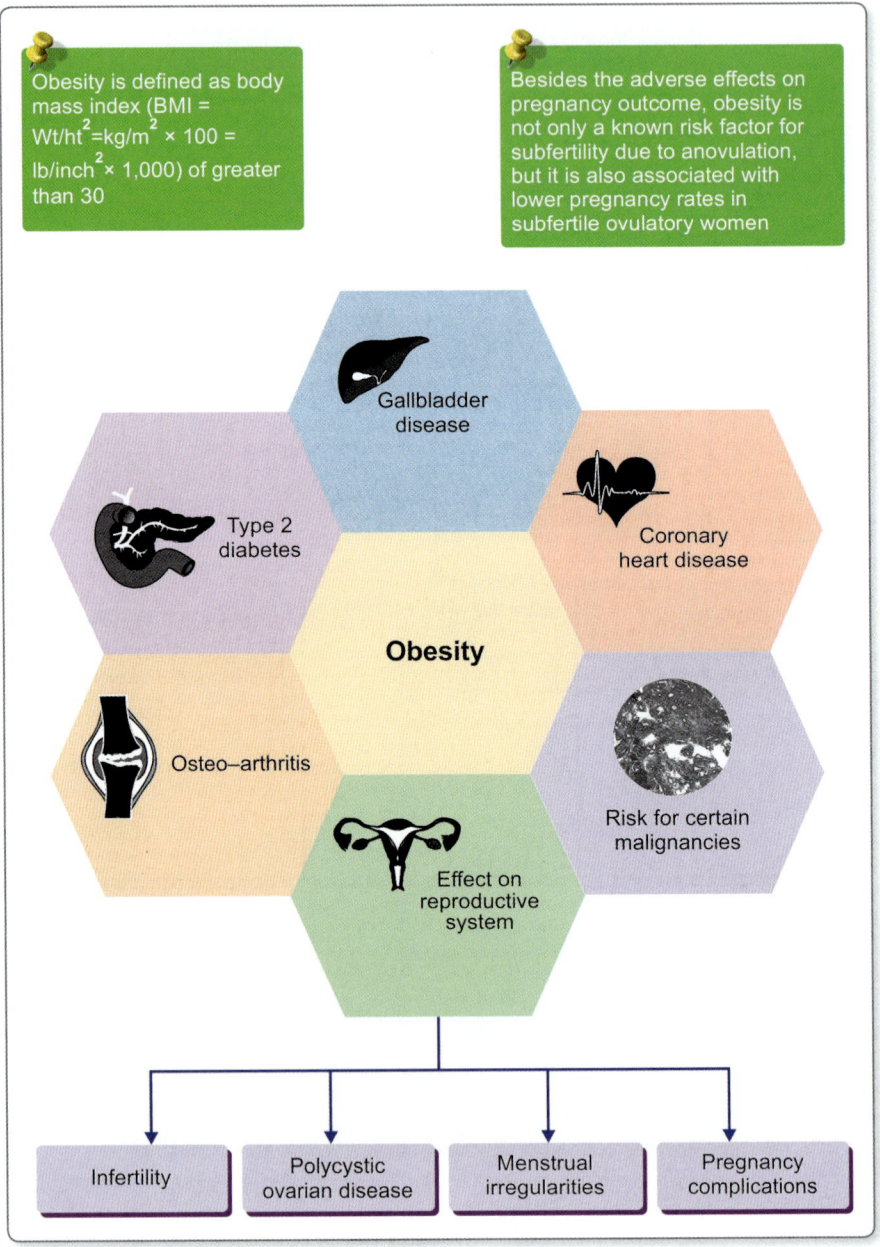

Flow Chart 24.1   Potential complications of obesity

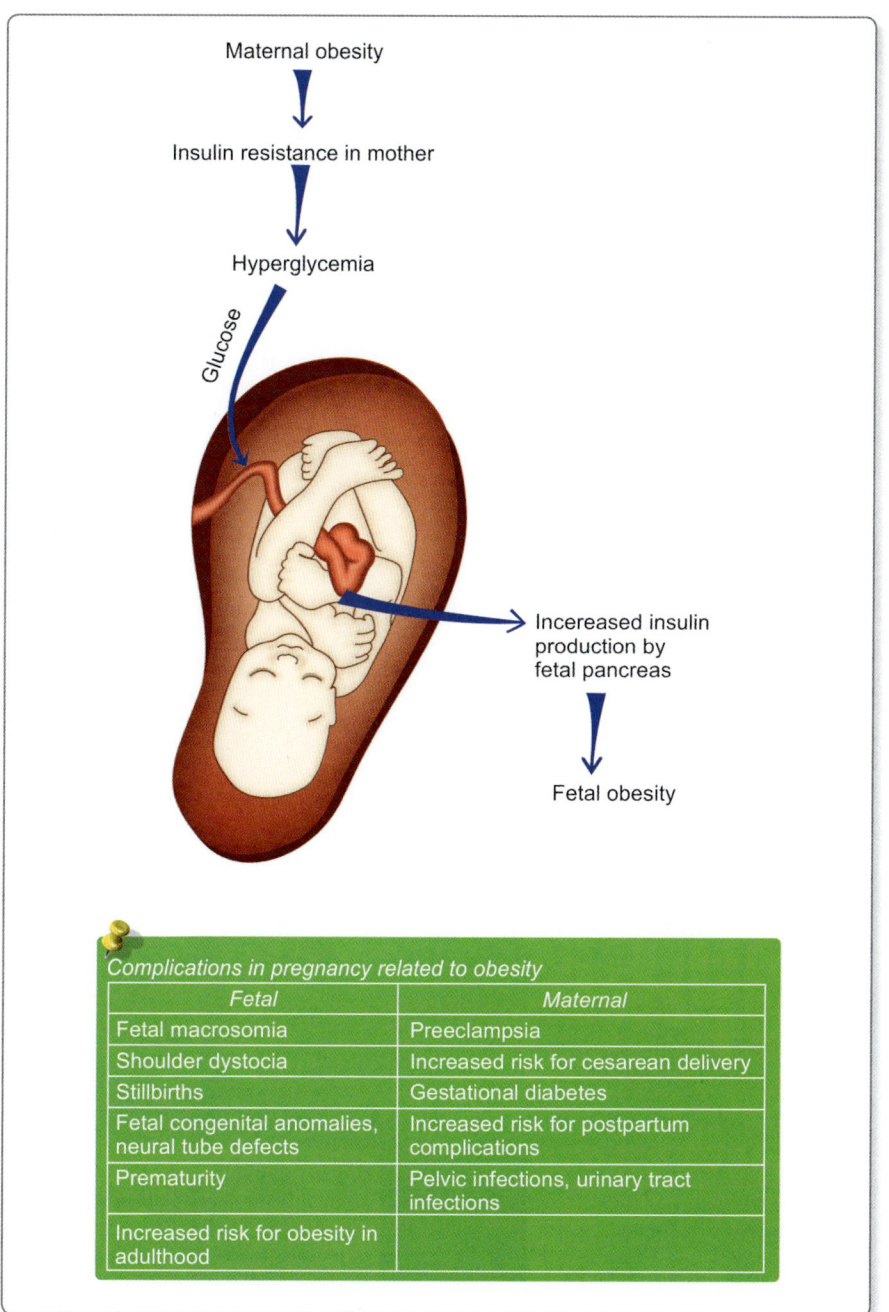

Flow Chart 24.2 Maternal obesity resulting in the development of fetal obesity

OBSTETRICS

Section 5: Postnatal Period

- **Chapter 25** — Postpartum Hemorrhage
- **Chapter 26** — Amniotic Fluid Embolism

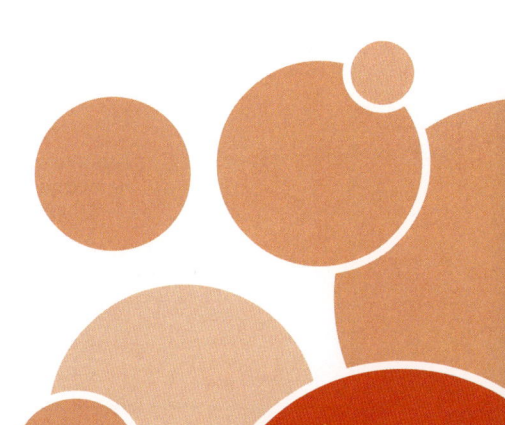

25 Postpartum Hemorrhage

Definition
Postpartum hemorrhage (PPH) can be defined as blood loss, estimated to be greater than 500 mL, occurring from the genital tract within 24 hours of delivery until 6 weeks postpartum. PPH can be of two types: primary and secondary.

WHO has defined postpartum hemorrhage as blood loss of 500 mL or more per vaginum during the first 24 hours after the vaginal delivery of the baby or blood loss of more than 1000 mL at the time of cesarean delivery.

Definition of postpartum hemorrhage

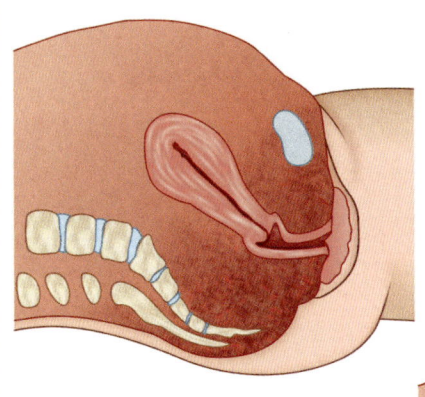
Normal postpartum patient with contracted uterus preventing hemorrhage

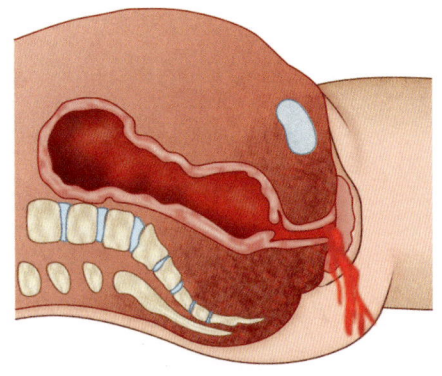
Uterine atony allows hemorrhage to flow into the uterus

Mechanism of bleeding in an atonic uterus

Various oxytocics used for controlling postpartum hemorrhage

Drug	Dosage	Side effects	Contraindications
Oxytocin 20 IU in 1 L of saline may be Water intoxication and nausea Nil	20 IU in 1 L of saline may be infused intravenously at a rate of 125 mL per hour	Water intoxication and nausea at high dosage	Nil
Methylergometrine (methergine)	0.25 mg intramuscularly or intravenously	Nausea, vomiting, hypertension, retained placenta, if given before placental separation, occurs	Hypertension, heart disease
Carboprost (15-methyl PGF2α)	250 µg given as intramuscular injection every 15 minutes for a maximum of eight doses	Diarrhea, vomiting, flushing, pyrexia, hypertension, bronchoconstriction, etc.	Significant pulmonary, cardiac, hepatic or renal disease
Misoprostol	600-1,000 µg per rectum or orally. Dose and frequency has yet not been standardized	Diarrhea, pyrexia (> 40°)	Significant pulmonary, cardiac, hepatic or renal disease

Oxytocics used to control PPH

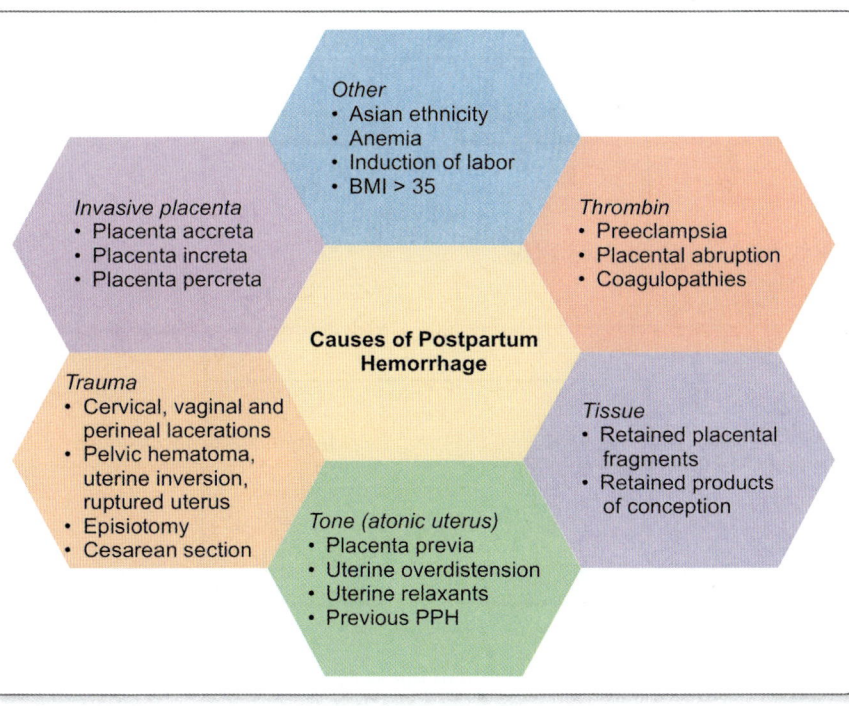

Various causes of postpartum hemorrhage

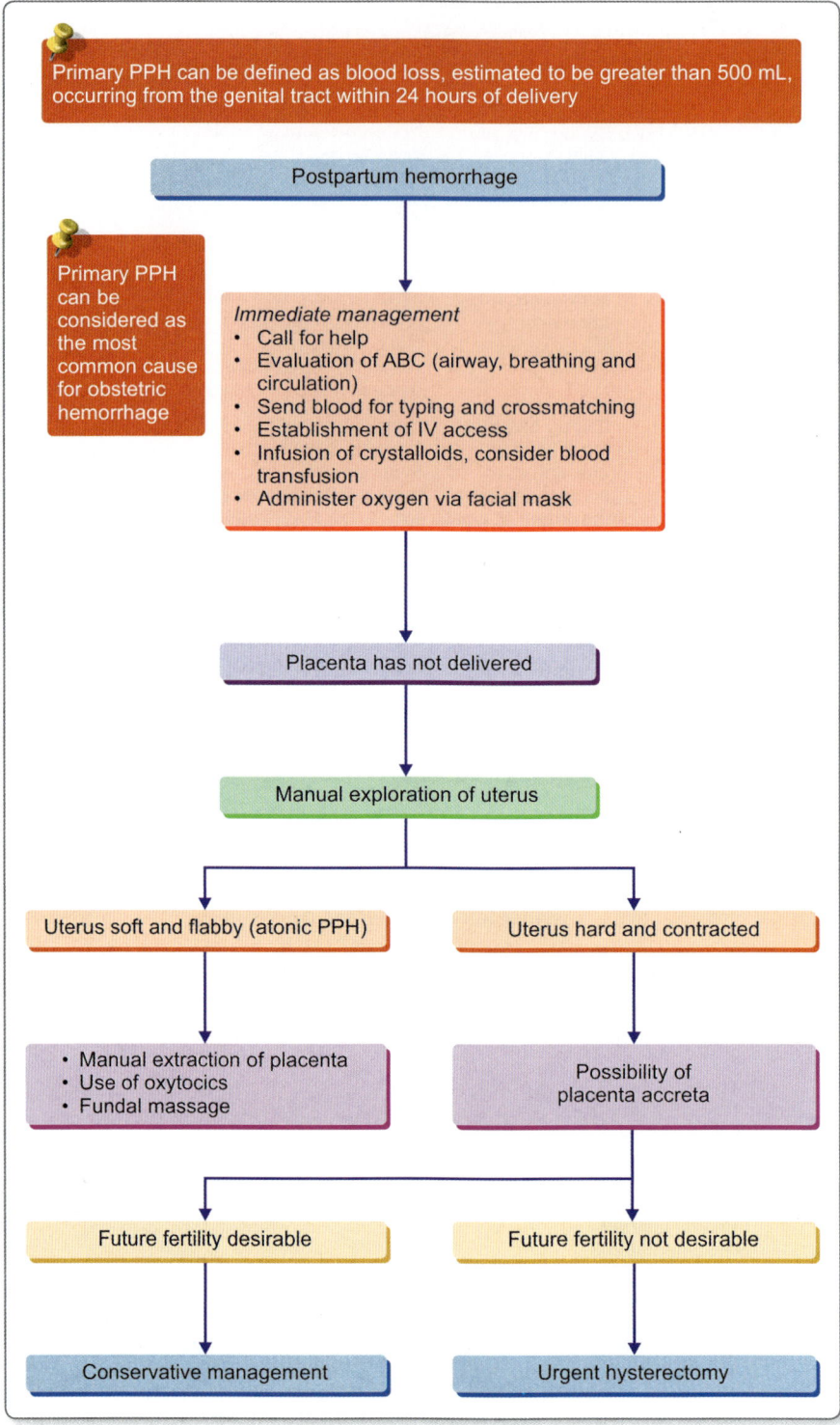

Flow Chart 25.1 Management of primary PPH, when placenta has not delivered

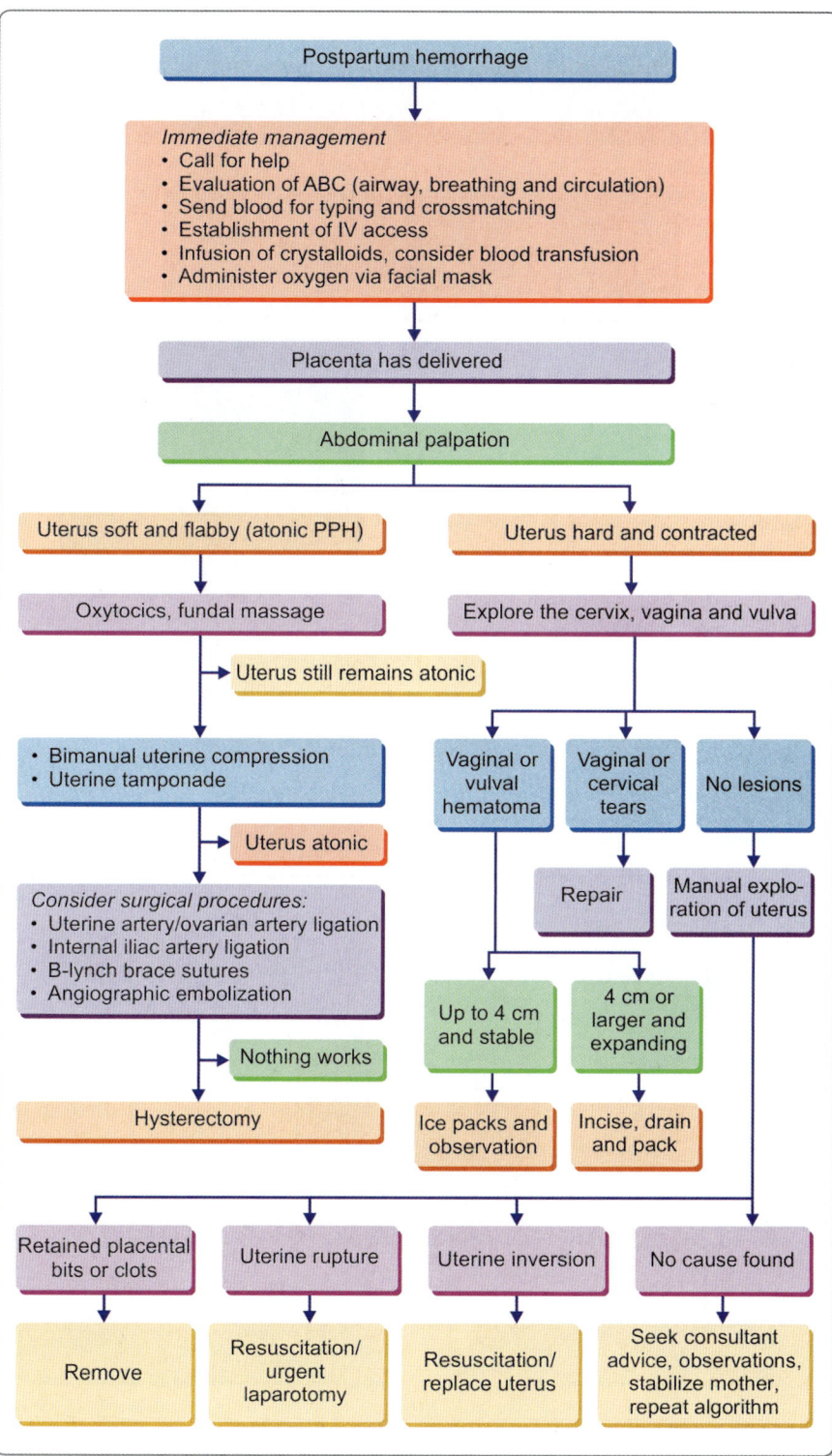

Flow Chart 25.2 Management of primary PPH, when placenta has delivered

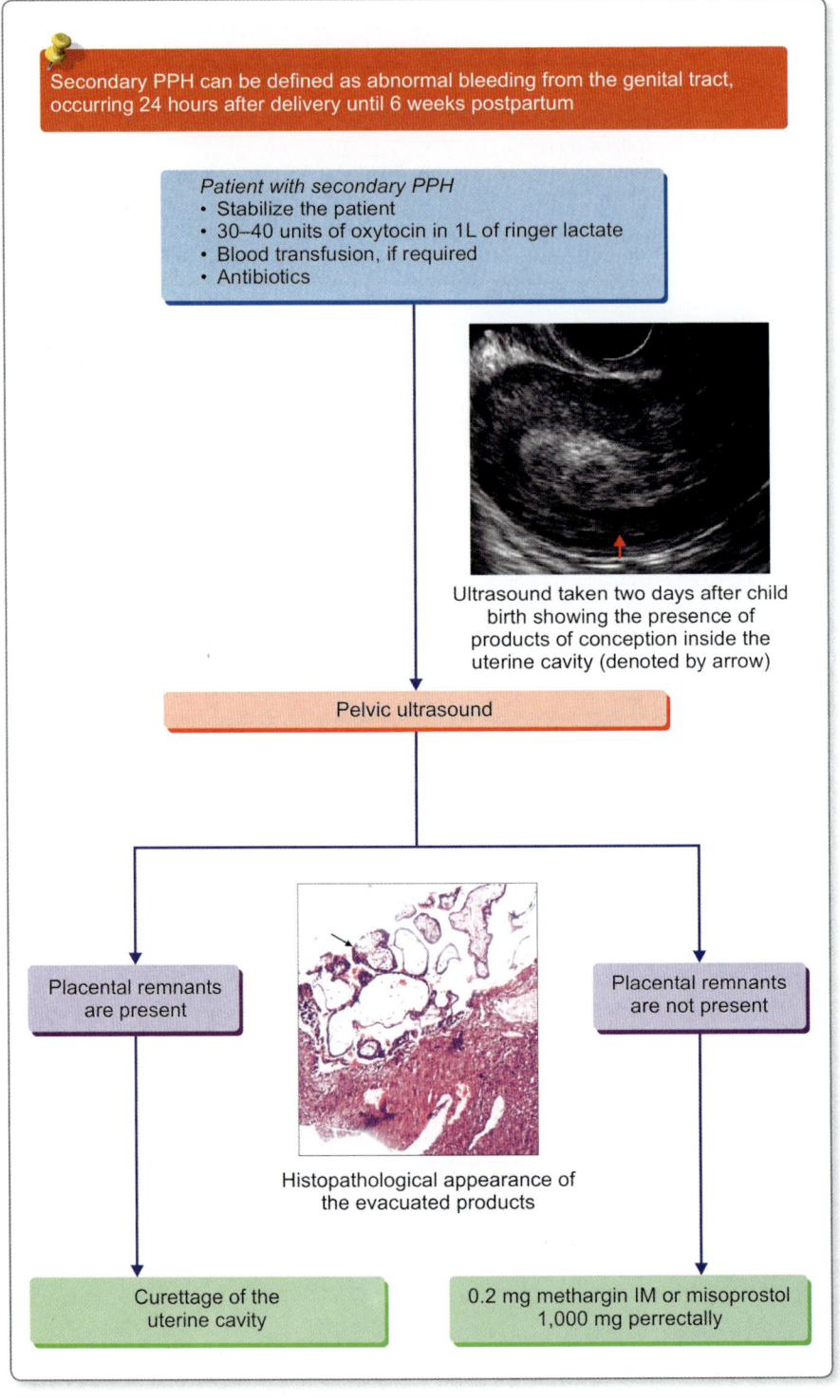

Flow Chart 25.3 Treatment of secondary PPH

26. Amniotic Fluid Embolism

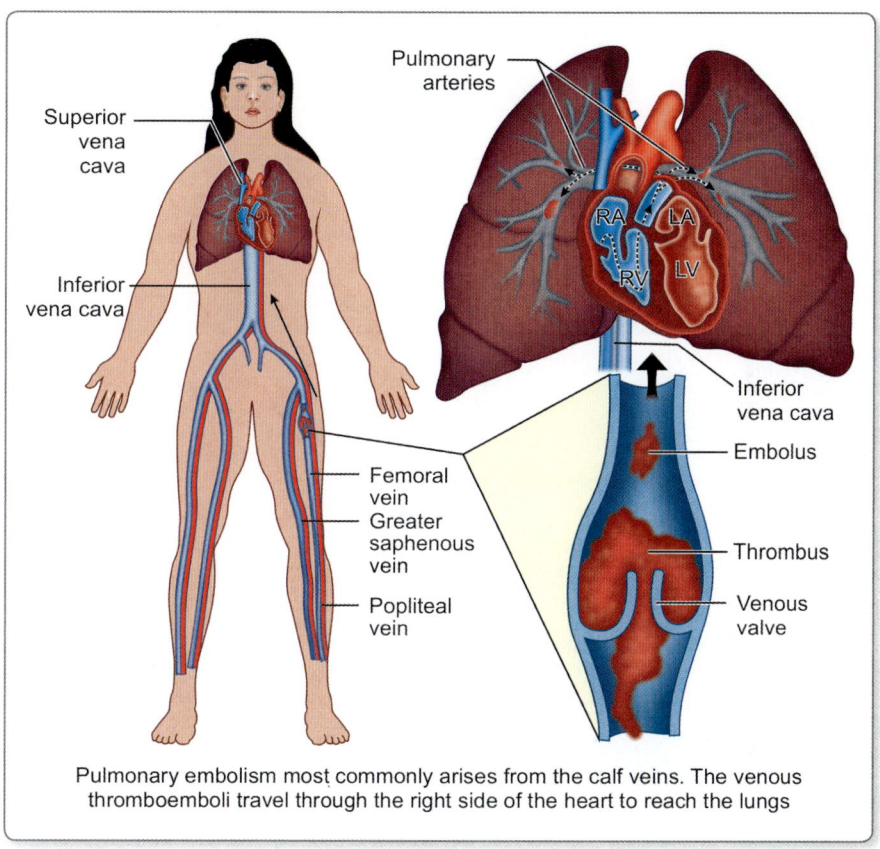

Pathogenesis of pulmonary embolism

Abbreviations: RA: Right atrium; RV: Right ventricle; LA: Left atrium; LV: Left ventricle

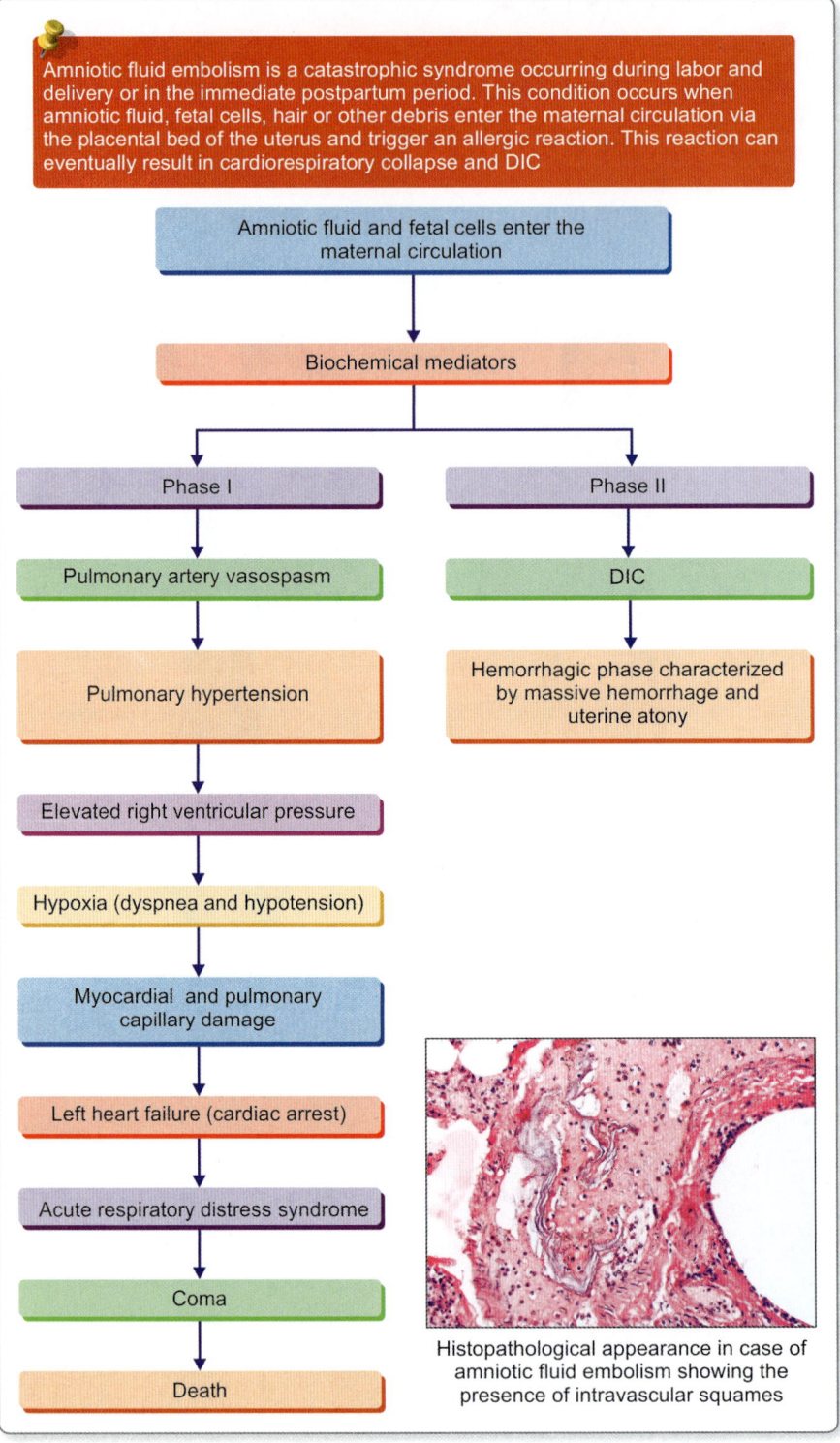

Flow Chart 26.1 Pathophysiology of amniotic fluid embolism

GYNECOLOGY

Section 6

General

Chapter 27 Normal Gynecological Examination

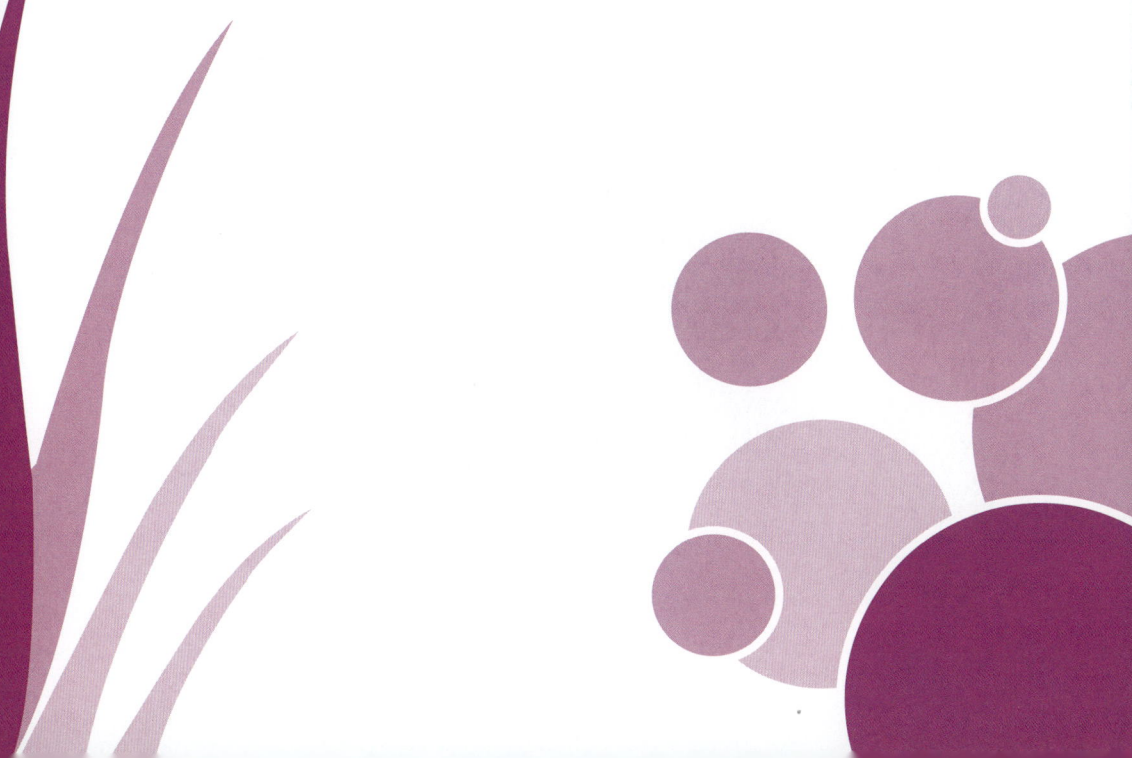

27 Normal Gynecological Examination

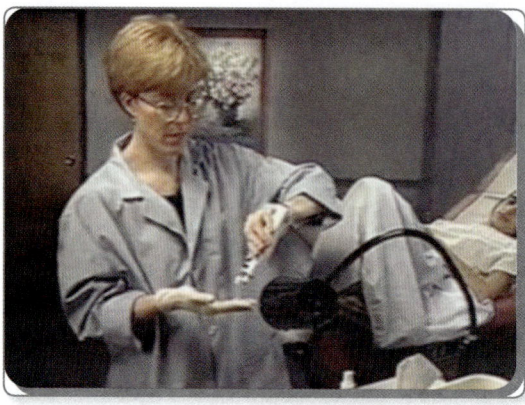

Use of a water-based non-greasy lubricant before starting vaginal examination

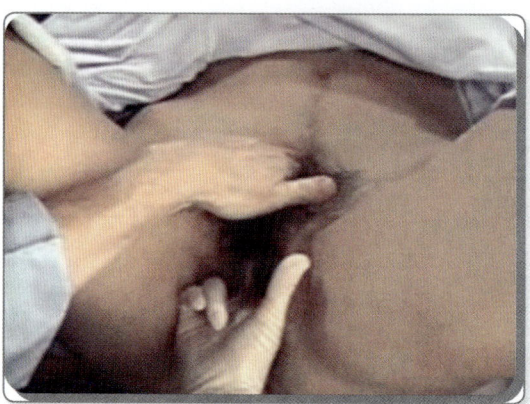

Bimanual vaginal examination

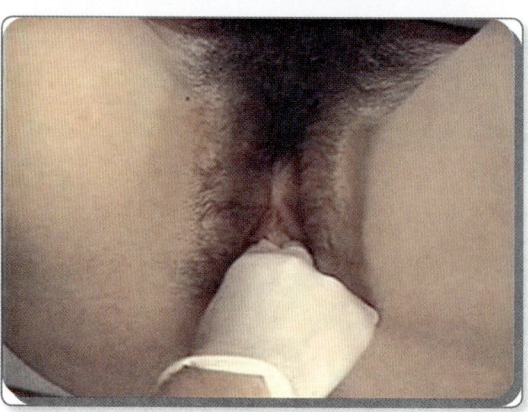

Two finger vaginal examination

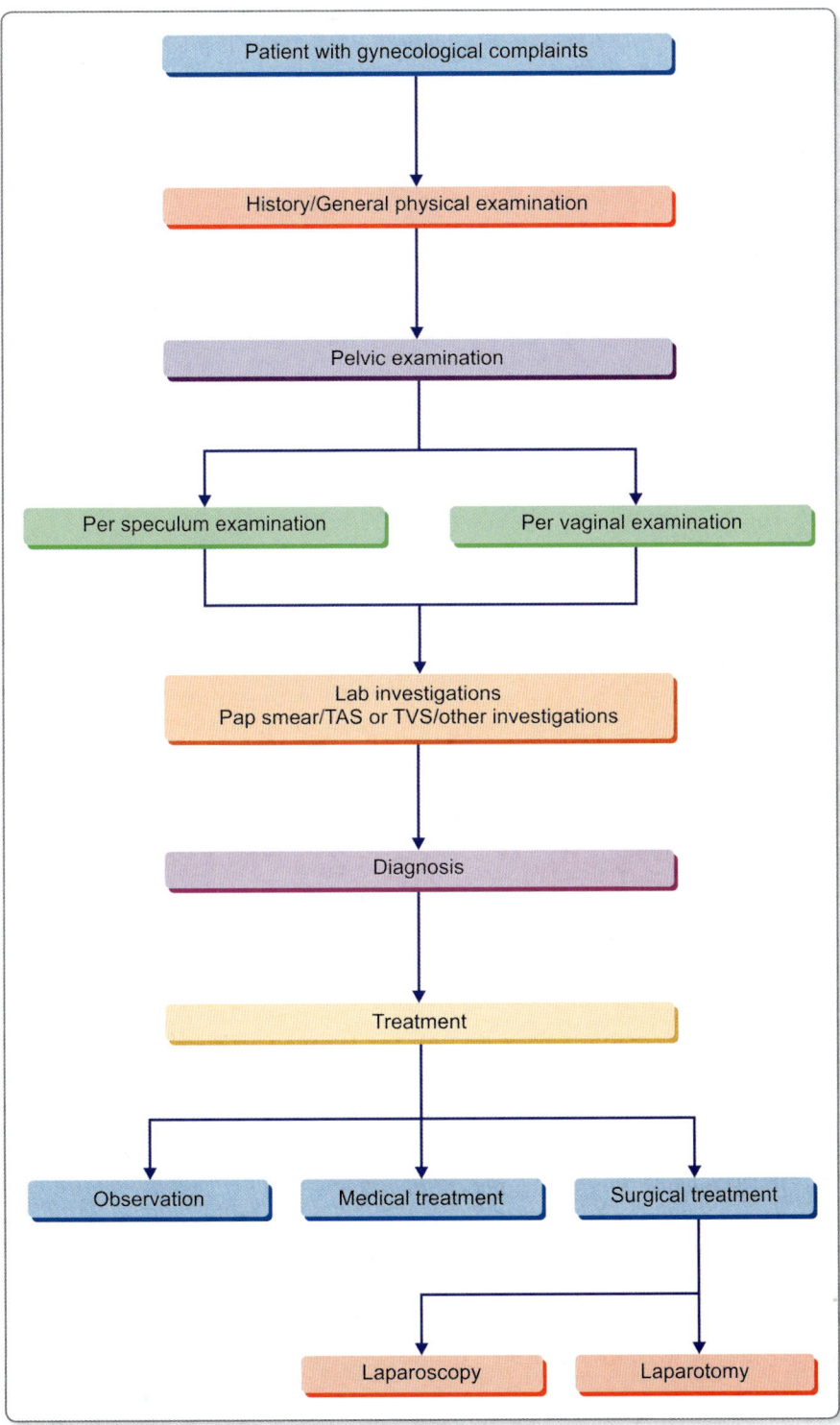

Flow Chart 27.1 Management of a patient presenting with gynecological complaints

GYNECOLOGY

Section 7

Abnormalities in Menstruation

Chapter 28   Abnormal Uterine Bleeding Due to Endometrial Cancer

Chapter 29   Dysfunctional Uterine Bleeding

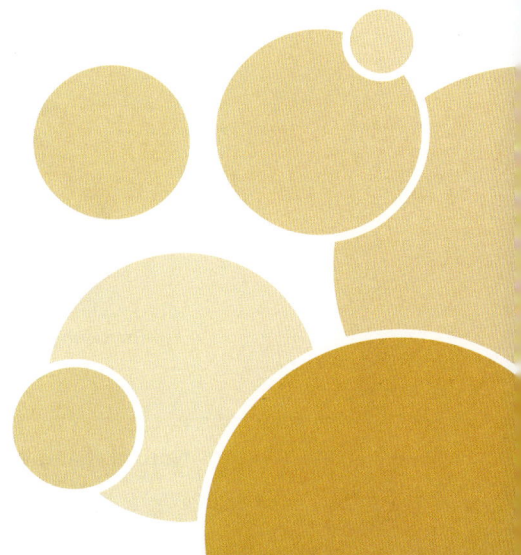

28 Abnormal Uterine Bleeding Due to Endometrial Cancer

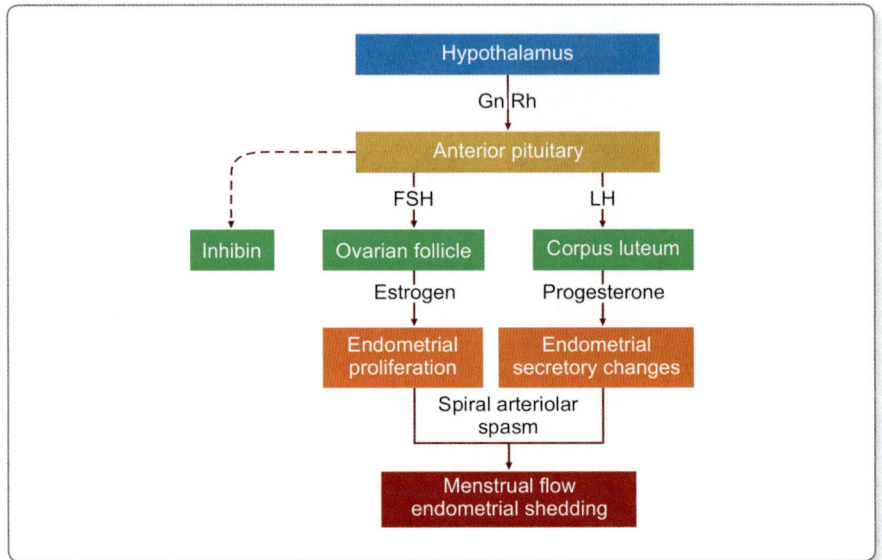

Normal pathophysiology of menstruation

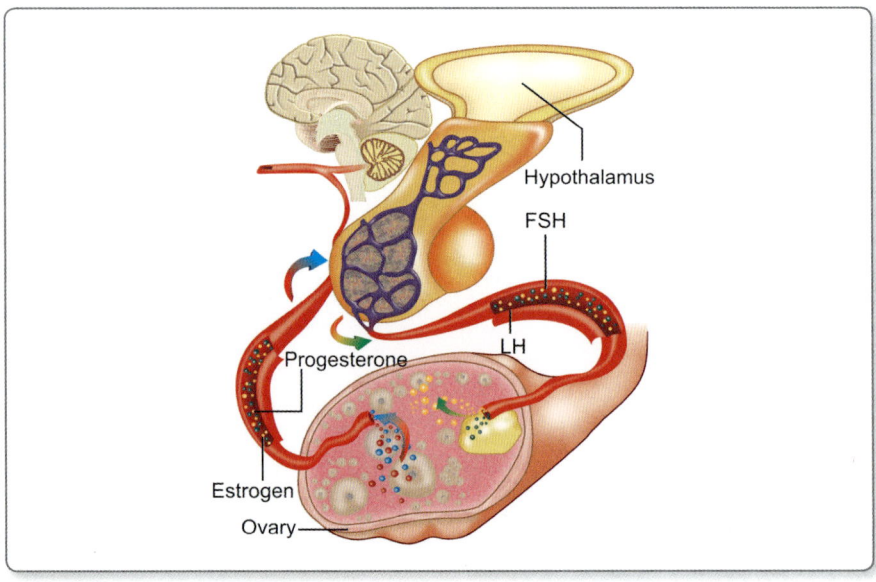

Normal changes occurring in the hypothalamus and pituitary resulting in menstrual cycle

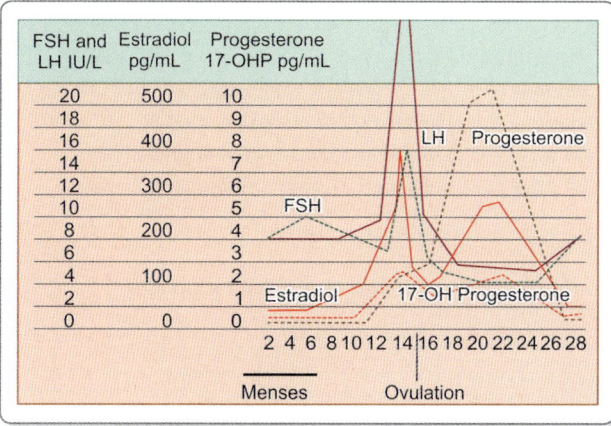

Levels of various hormones during different phases of menstrual cycle

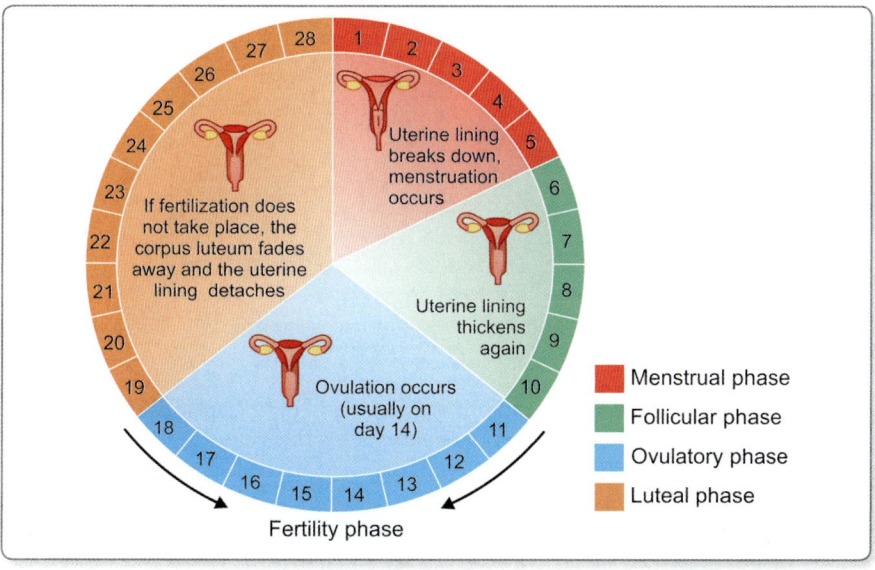

Correlation of various phases of menstrual cycle with fertility

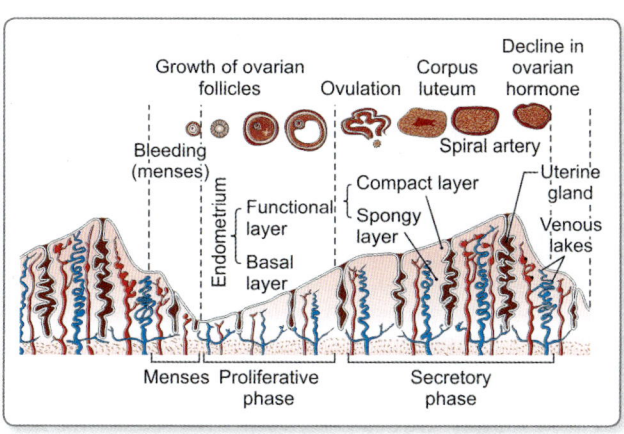

Phases of endometrium during various stages of menstrual cycle

Parameters for normal and abnormal menstrual blood loss

Parameters	Normal	Abnormal
Duration	4–6 days	Less than 2 or more than 7 days
Volume	30–80 mL	Less than 30 mL or more than 80 mL
Interval	24–35 days	Less than 21 days or more than 35 days

Different parameters for normal and abnormal blood loss

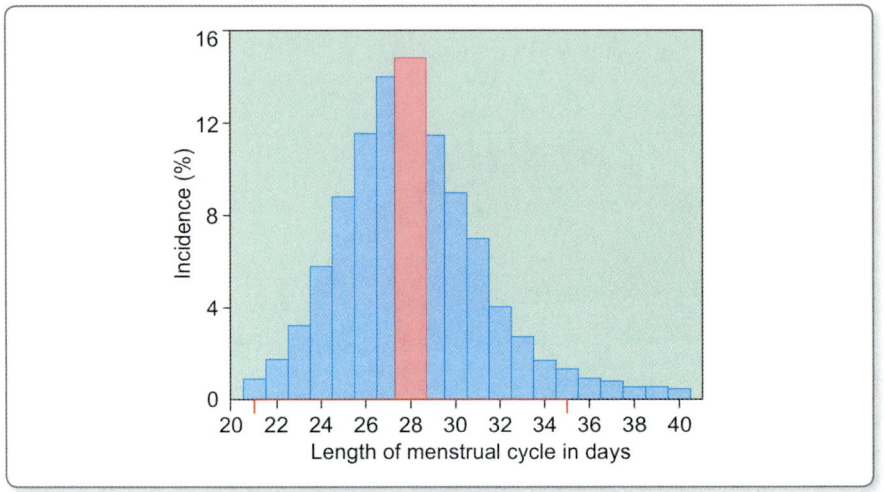

Criteria for abnormal bleeding: in most women, normal menstrual cycles occur at every 28 ± 7 days

Terms used for describing AUB

Term	Definition
Menorrhagia	Prolonged or excessive menstrual blood loss (> 80 mL) at regular intervals
Polymenorrhea	Regular bleeding at intervals of less than 21 days
Oligomenorrhea	Infrequent menstruation at intervals greater than every 35 days
Amenorrhea	No uterine bleeding for at least 6 months
Intermenstrual bleeding (spotting)	Episodes of uterine bleeding of varying amounts occurring between the regular menstrual periods
Menometrorrhagia	Combination of both menorrhagia and metrorrhagia, associated with prolonged or excessive bleeding (> 80 mL) at irregular intervals
Metrorrhagia	Irregular, frequent uterine bleeding of varying amounts, but not excessive at irregular intervals
Hypomenorrhea	Scanty menstruation

Term used for describing abnormal uterine bleeding

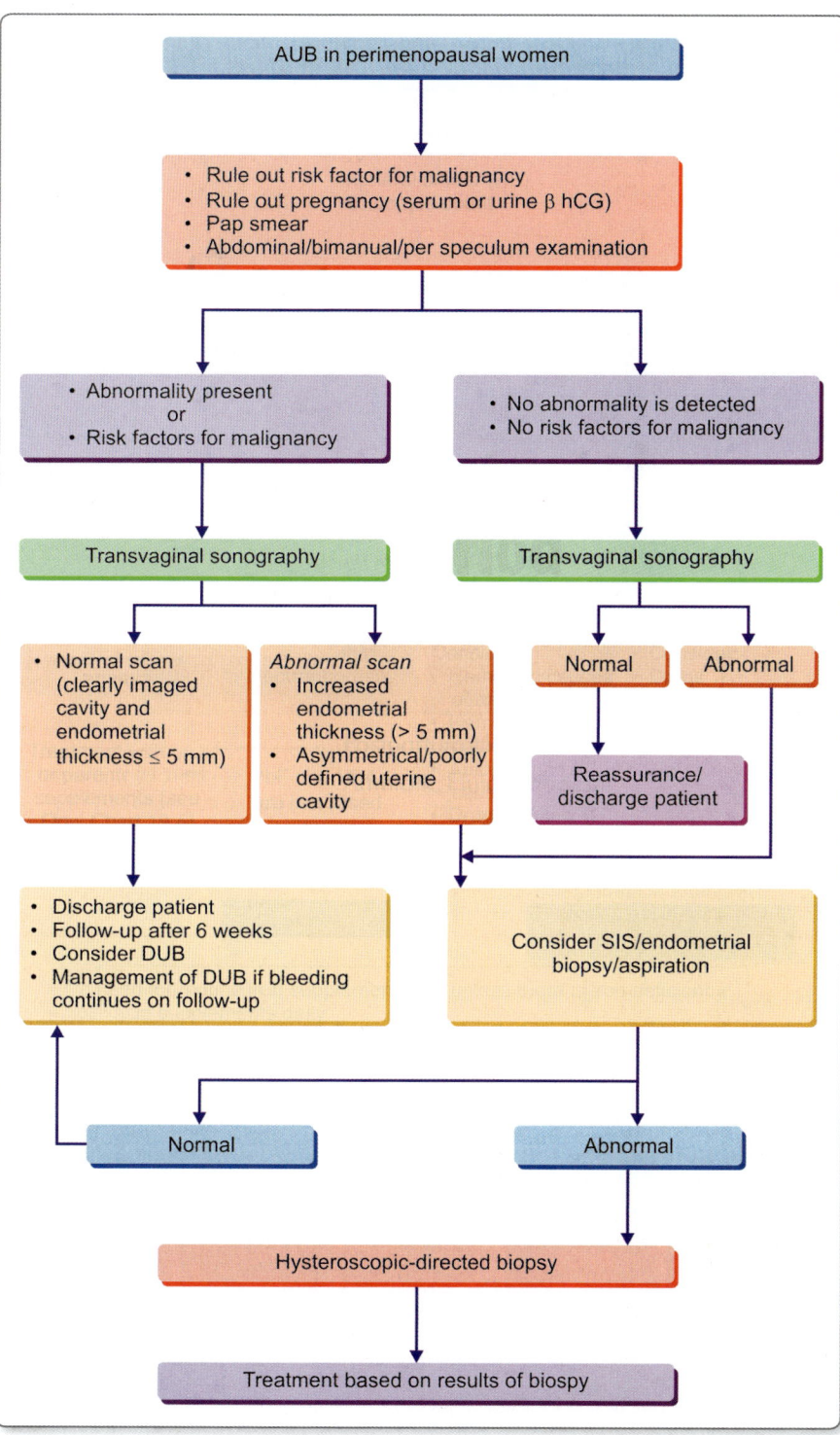

Flow Chart 28.1 Management of AUB (perimenopausal women)

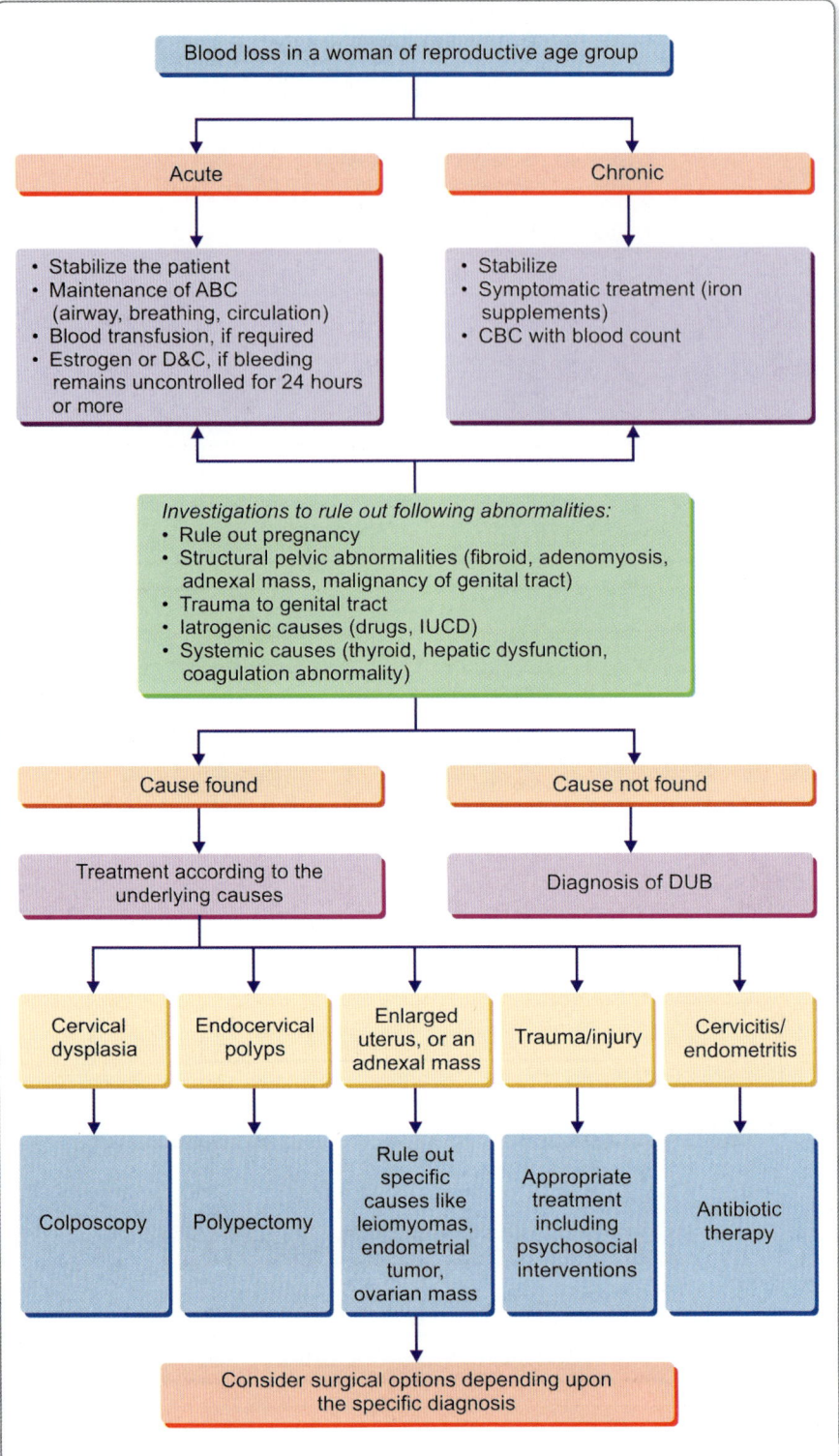

Flow Chart 28.2 Management of AUB (women in reproductive age group)

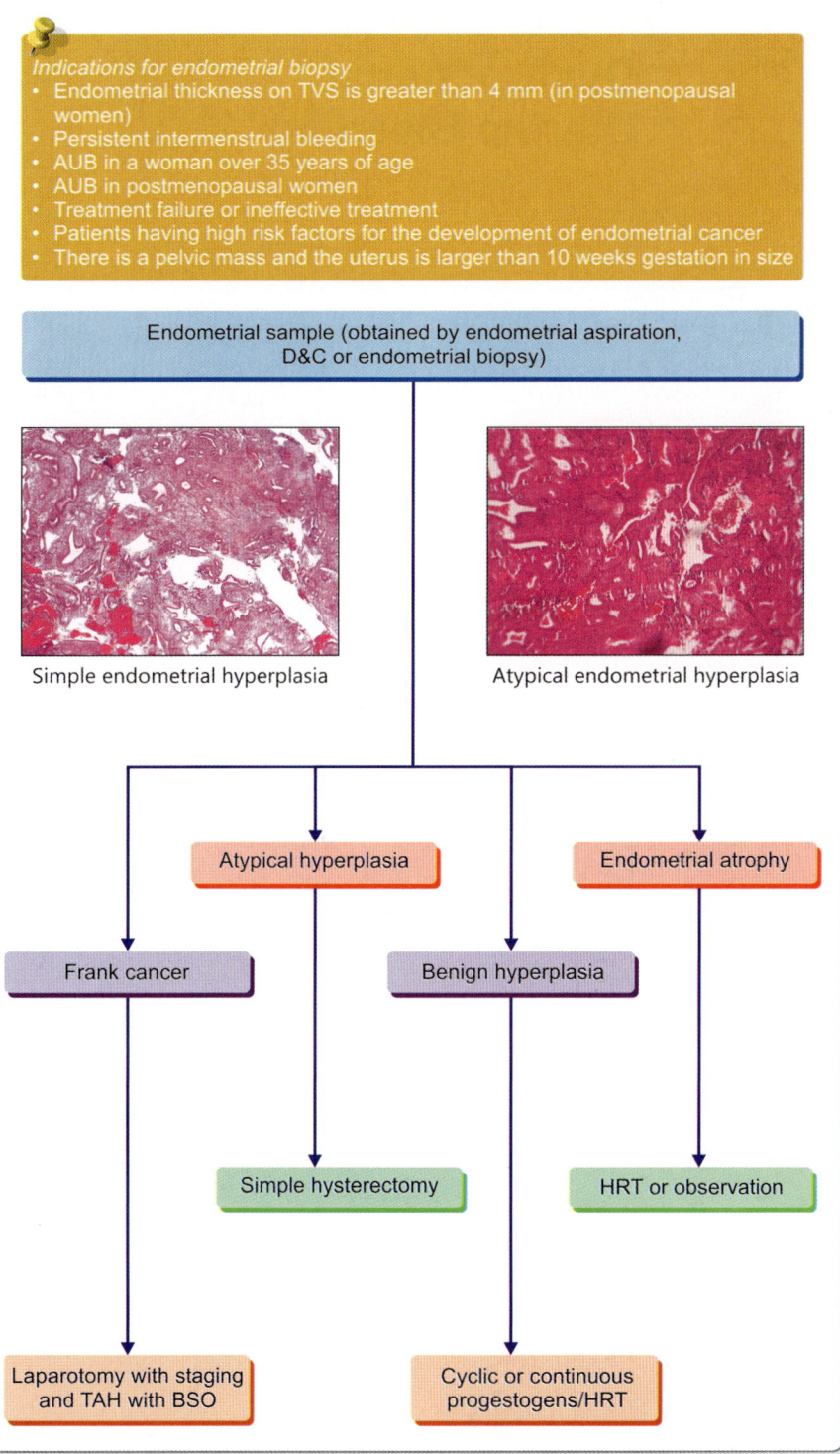

Flow Chart 28.3 Management of endometrial hyperplasia

29 Dysfunctional Uterine Bleeding

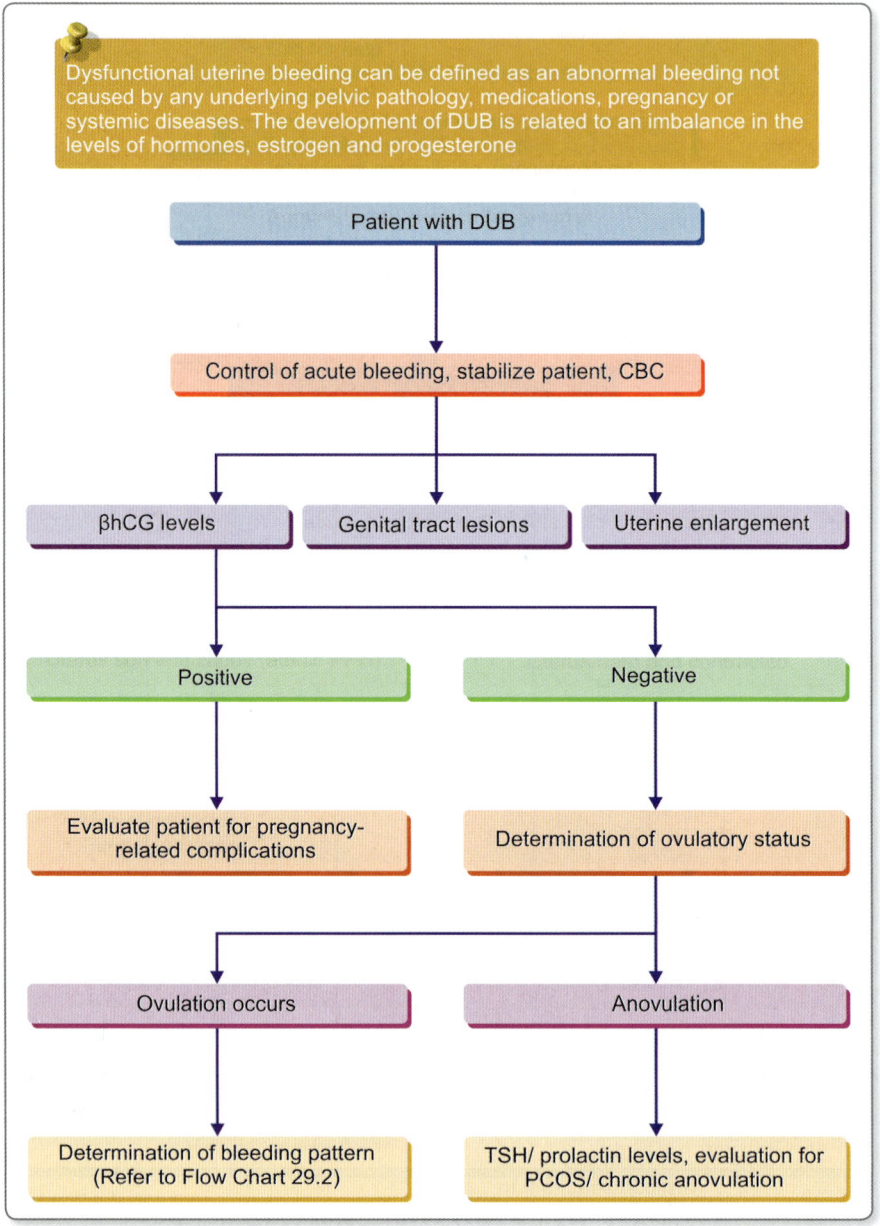

Flow Chart 29.1 Treatment of DUB in a woman of reproductive age group

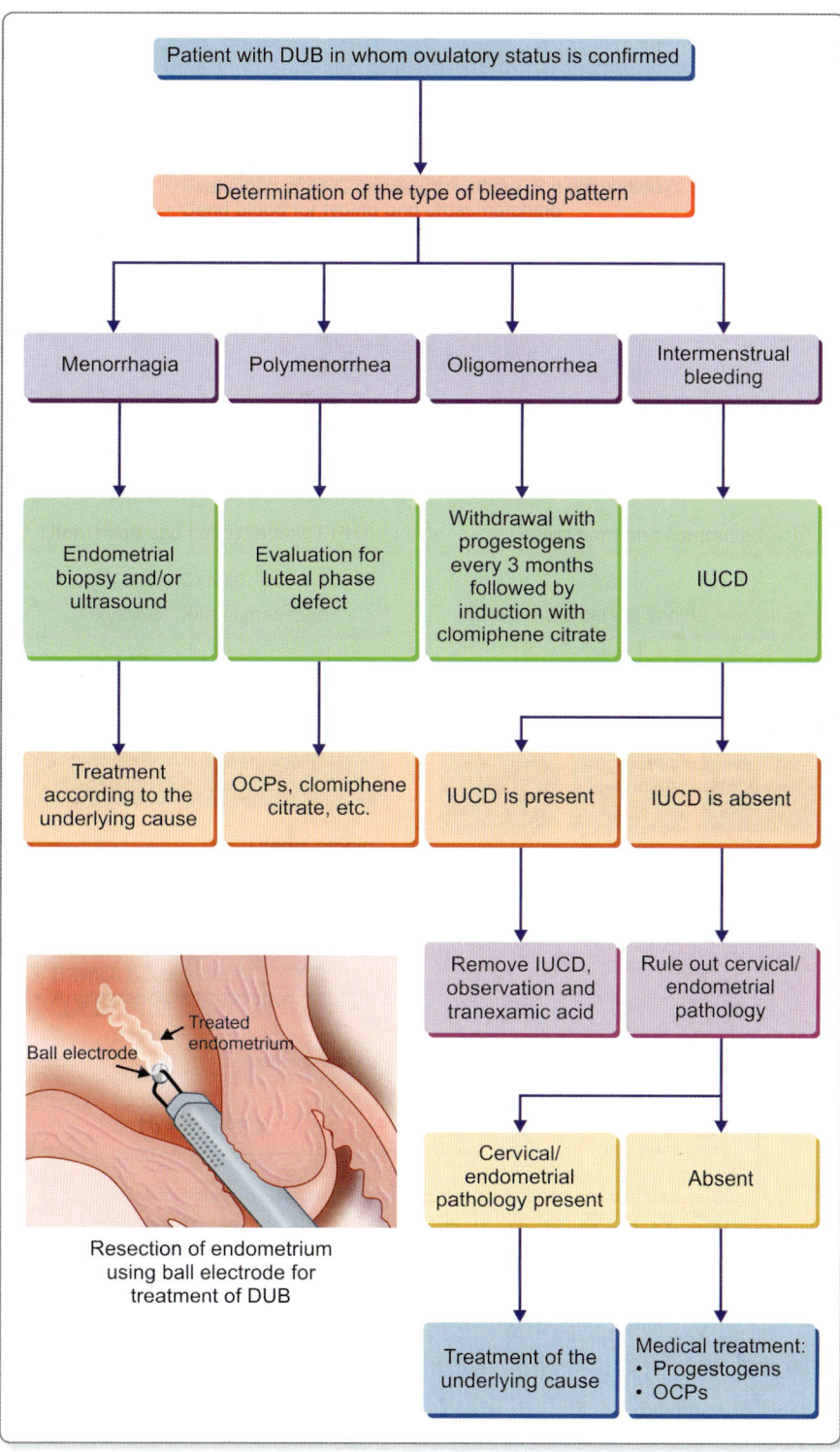

Flow Chart 29.2 Treatment of DUB in a woman of reproductive age in whom ovulatory status is confirmed

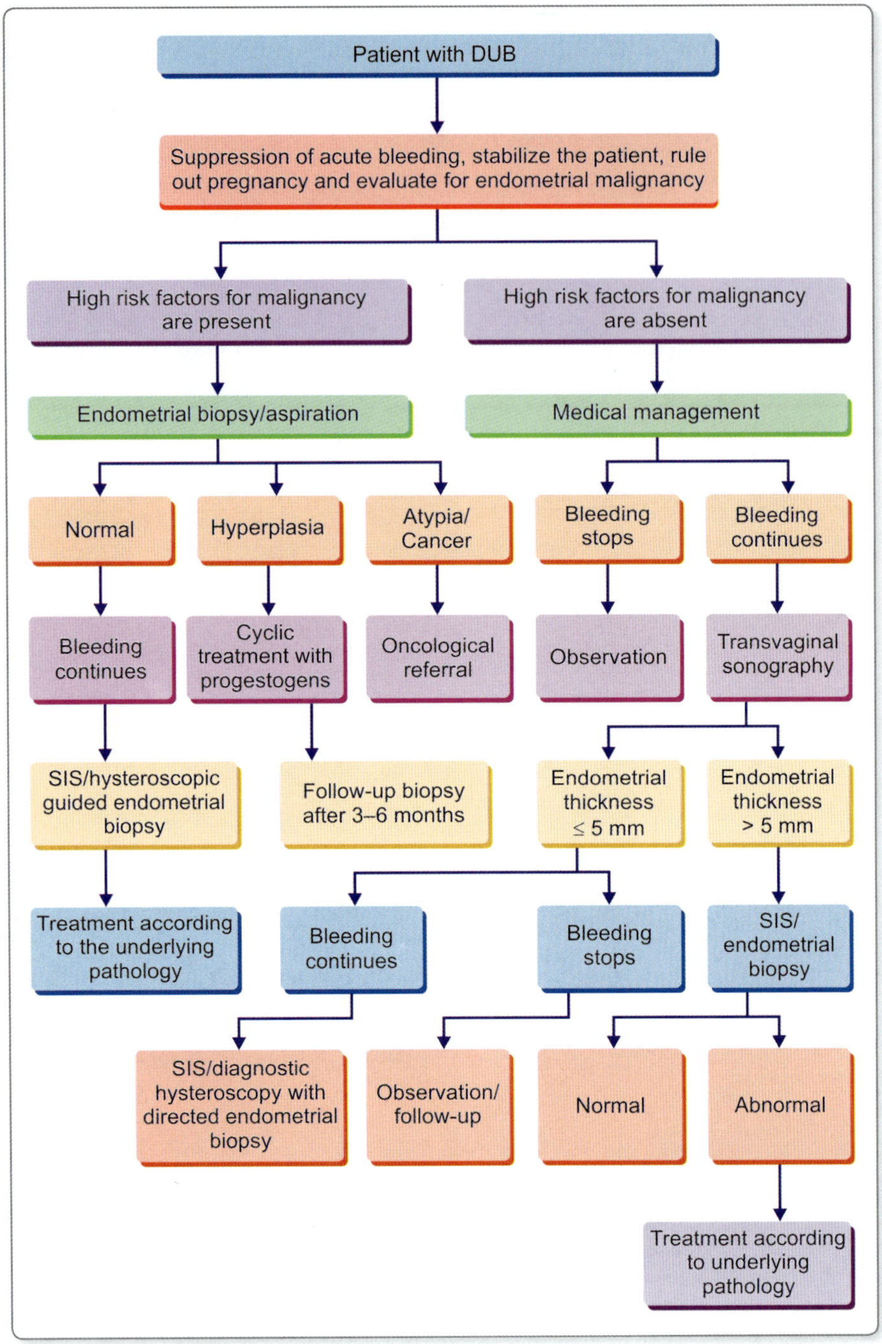

Flow Chart 29.3 Treatment of DUB in perimenopausal women

GYNECOLOGY

Section 8

Benign Masses

Chapter 30 Leiomyomas

30 Leiomyomas

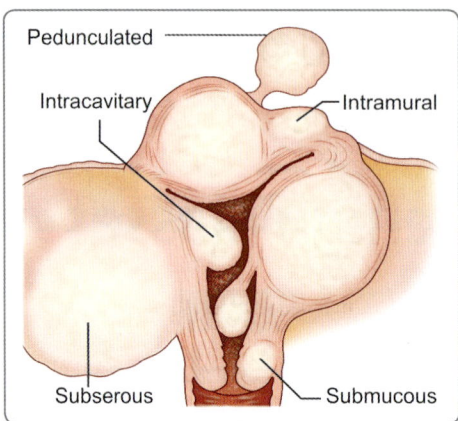

Diagram showing different types of leiomyomas (fibroids)

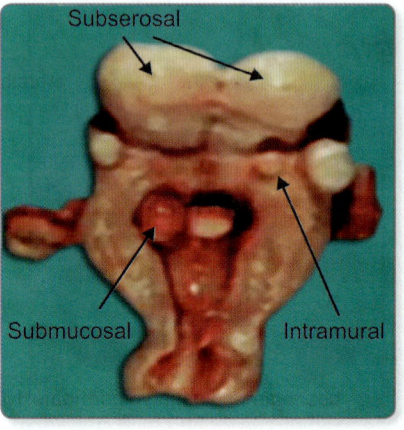

Different types of leiomyomas as observed in the hysterectomy specimen

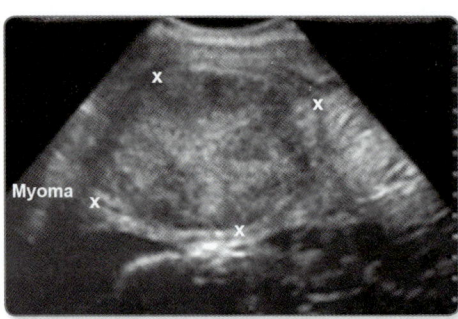

Presence of an intramural fibroid on ultrasound

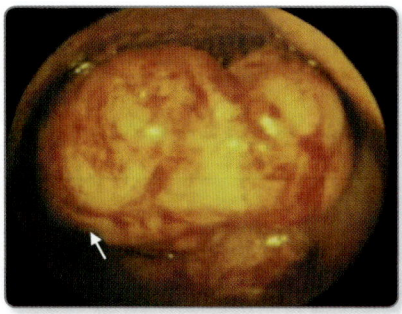

Appearance of submucosal myoma on hysteroscopy (indicated by an arrow)

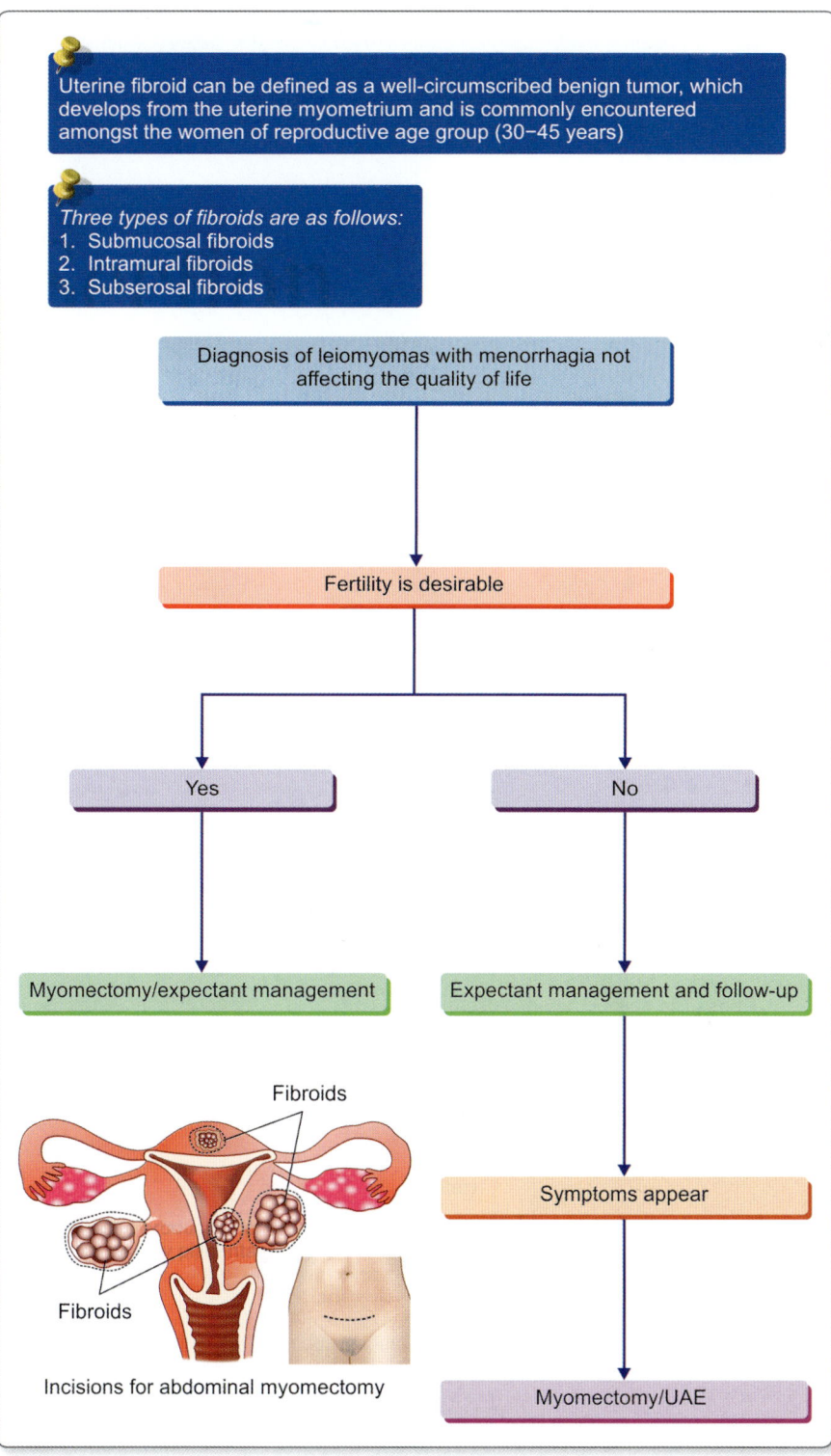

Flow Chart 30.1 Management plan of a patient with fibroids, presenting with menorrhagia not affecting the quality of life

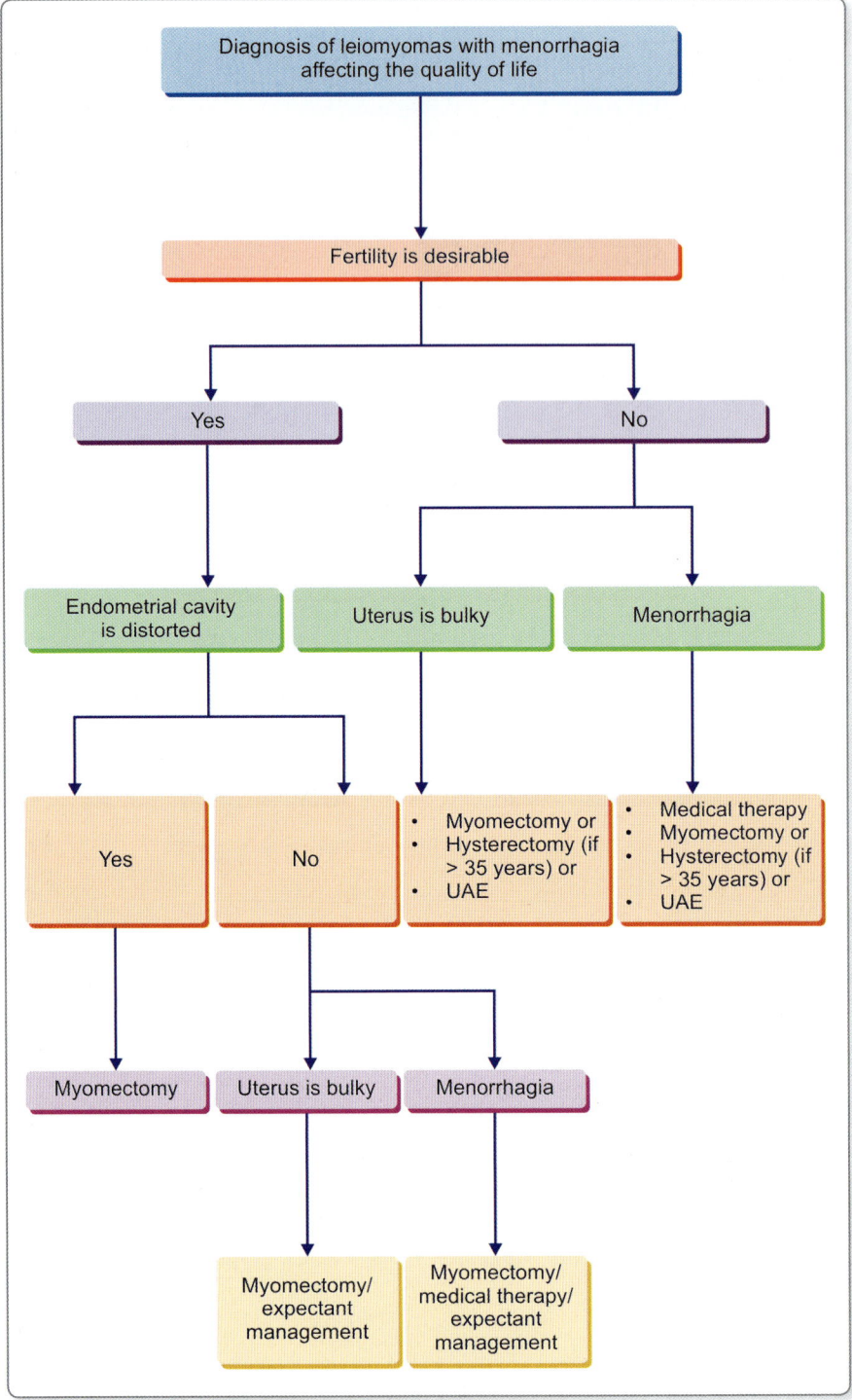

Flow Chart 30.2 Management plan of a patient with fibroids, presenting with menorrhagia affecting the quality of life

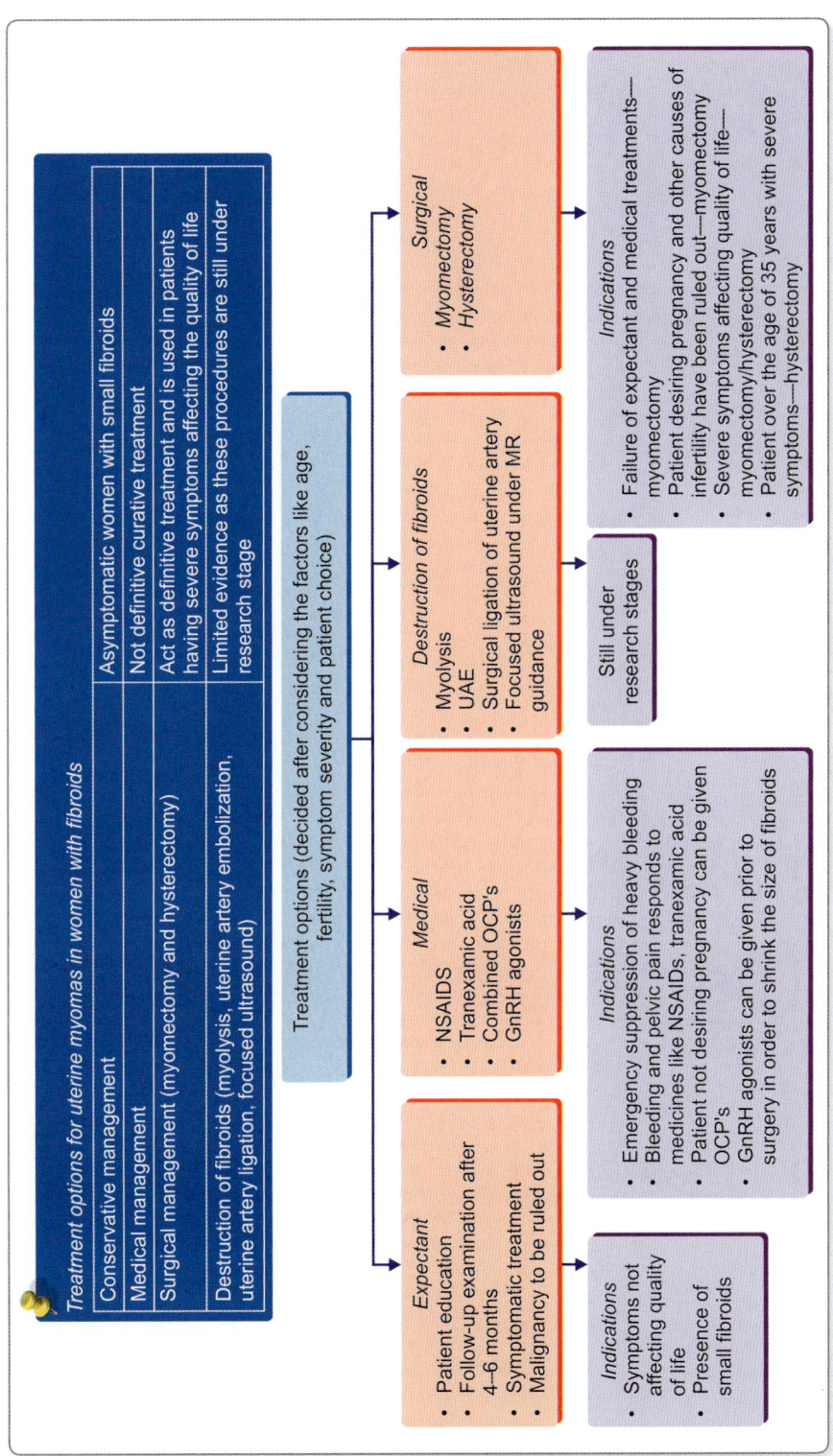

Flow Chart 30.3 Treatment options for a patient diagnosed with fibroids uterus

GYNECOLOGY

Section 9

Infections in Pregnancy

Chapter 31   Vaginal Discharge

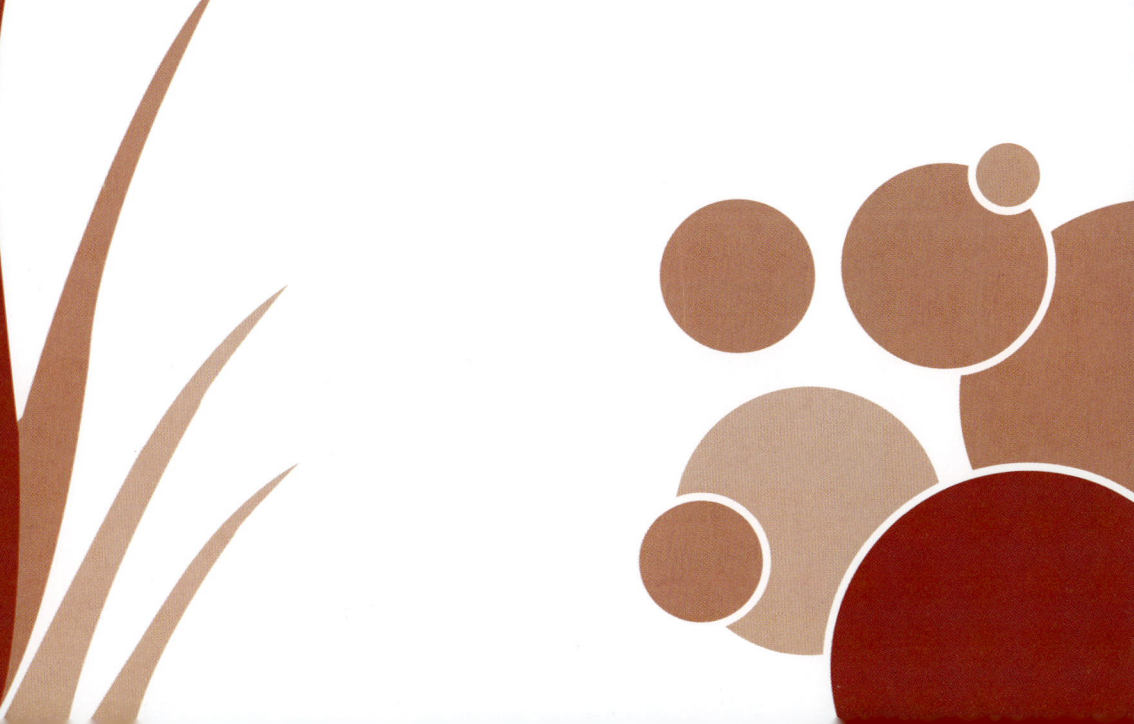

31 Vaginal Discharge

Features of the most common causes of vaginitis

Basis of diagnosis	Bacterial vaginosis	Vulvovaginal candidiasis	Trichomoniasis
Signs and symptoms	Thin, grayish to off-white colored discharge; unpleasant "fishy" odor, with odor especially increasing after sexual intercourse. The discharge is usually homogeneous and adheres to vaginal walls	Thick, white ("curd like") discharge with no odor	Copious, malodorous, yellow-green (or discolored) discharge, pruritus and vaginal irritation, dysuria, no symptoms in 20–50% of affected women
Physical examination	Normal appearance of vaginal tissues; grayish-white colored discharge may be adherent to the vaginal walls	Vulvar and vaginal erythema, edema and fissures. Thick, white discharge that adheres to vaginal walls	Vulvar and vaginal edema and erythema, "strawberry" cervix in up to 25% of affected women. Frothy, purulent discharge
Vaginal pH (normal ≤ 4.5)	Elevated (> 4.5)	Normal	Elevated (> 4.5)
Microscopic examination of wet-mount and KOH preparations of vaginal discharge	"Clue cells" (vaginal epithelial cells coated with coccobacilli), few lactobacilli, occasional motile, curved rods, belonging to *Mobiluncus* species	Pseudohyphae, mycelial tangles or budding yeast cells	Motile trichomonads and many polymorphonuclear cells
"Whiff" test (Normal = no odor)	Positive	Negative	Can be positive
Additional tests	Amsel's criteria is positive in nearly 90% of affected women with bacterial vaginosis	KOH microscopy, Gram stain, culture	DNA probe tests: Sensitivity of 90% and specificity of 99.8%. Culture: Sensitivity of 98% and specificity of 100%

Basic features of the most common causes vaginitis

Source: (1) Carr PL, Felsenstein D, Friedman RH. Evaluation and managment of vaginitis. J Gen Intern Med. 1998;13:335–46. (2) Sobel JD. Vaginitis. N Engl J Med. 1997;337:1896–903.

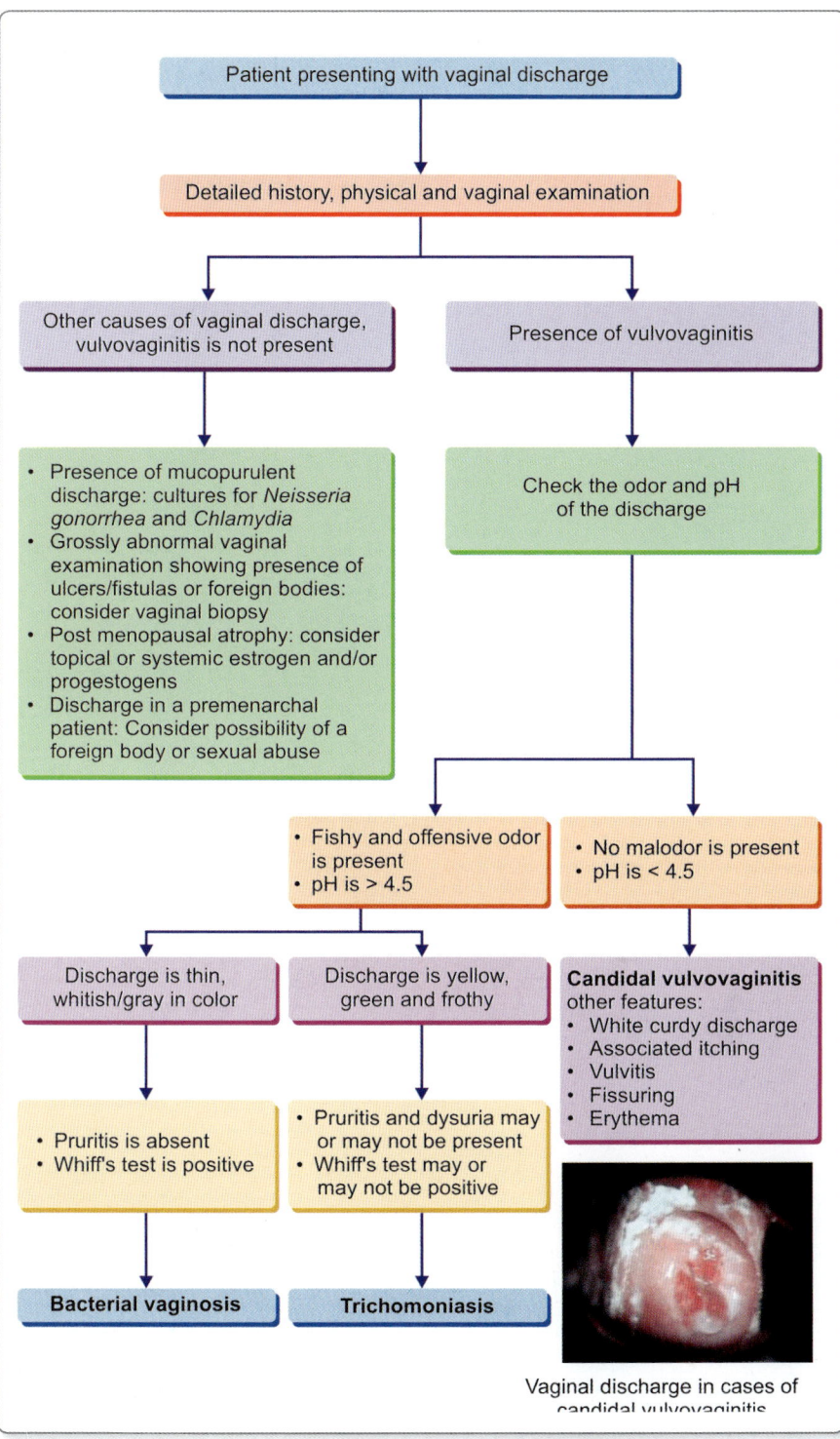

Flow Chart 31.1 Management plan for a patient presenting with vaginal discharge

GYNECOLOGY

Section 10

Malignancies of the Genital Tract

- **Chapter 32** Cervical Cancer
- **Chapter 33** Ovarian Neoplasms

32 Cervical Cancer

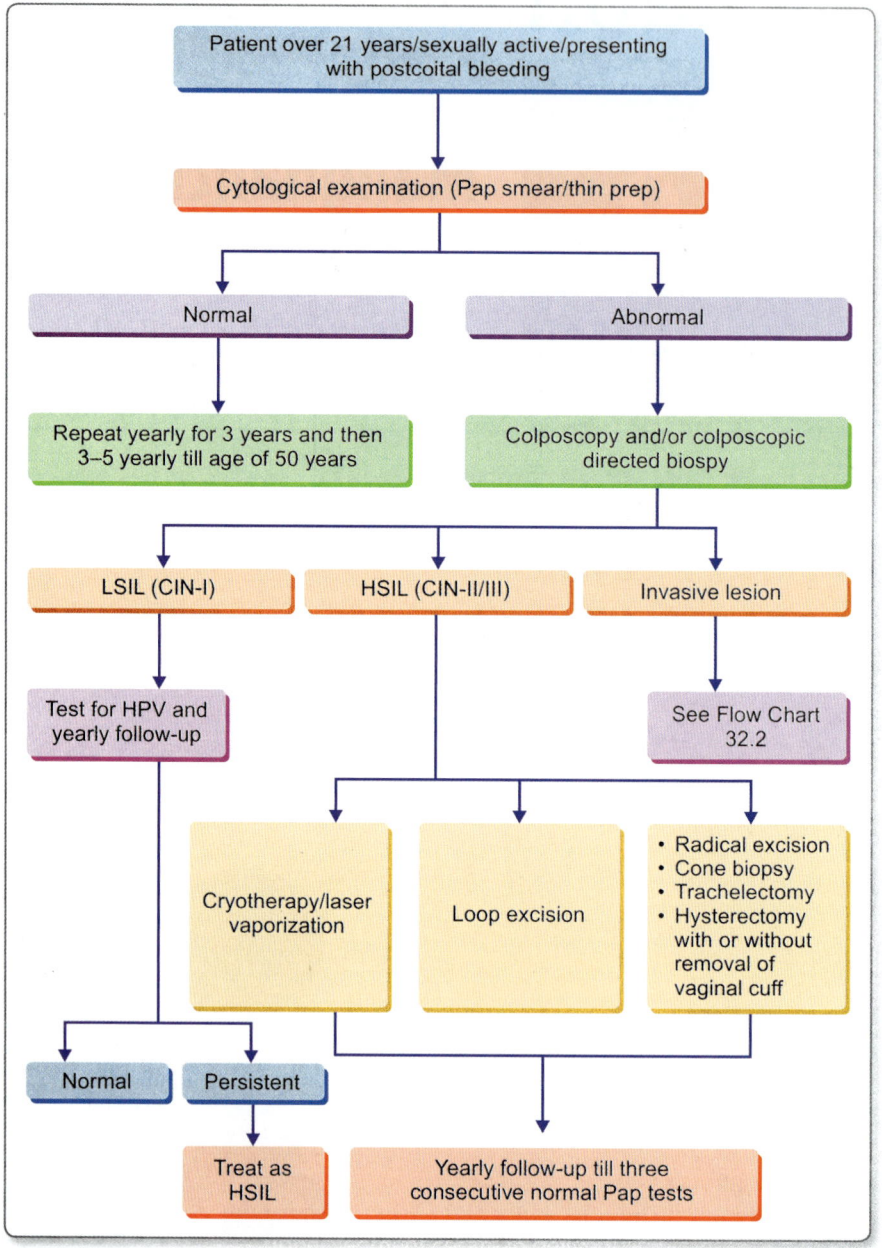

Flow Chart 32.1 Management of patients with preinvasive lesions

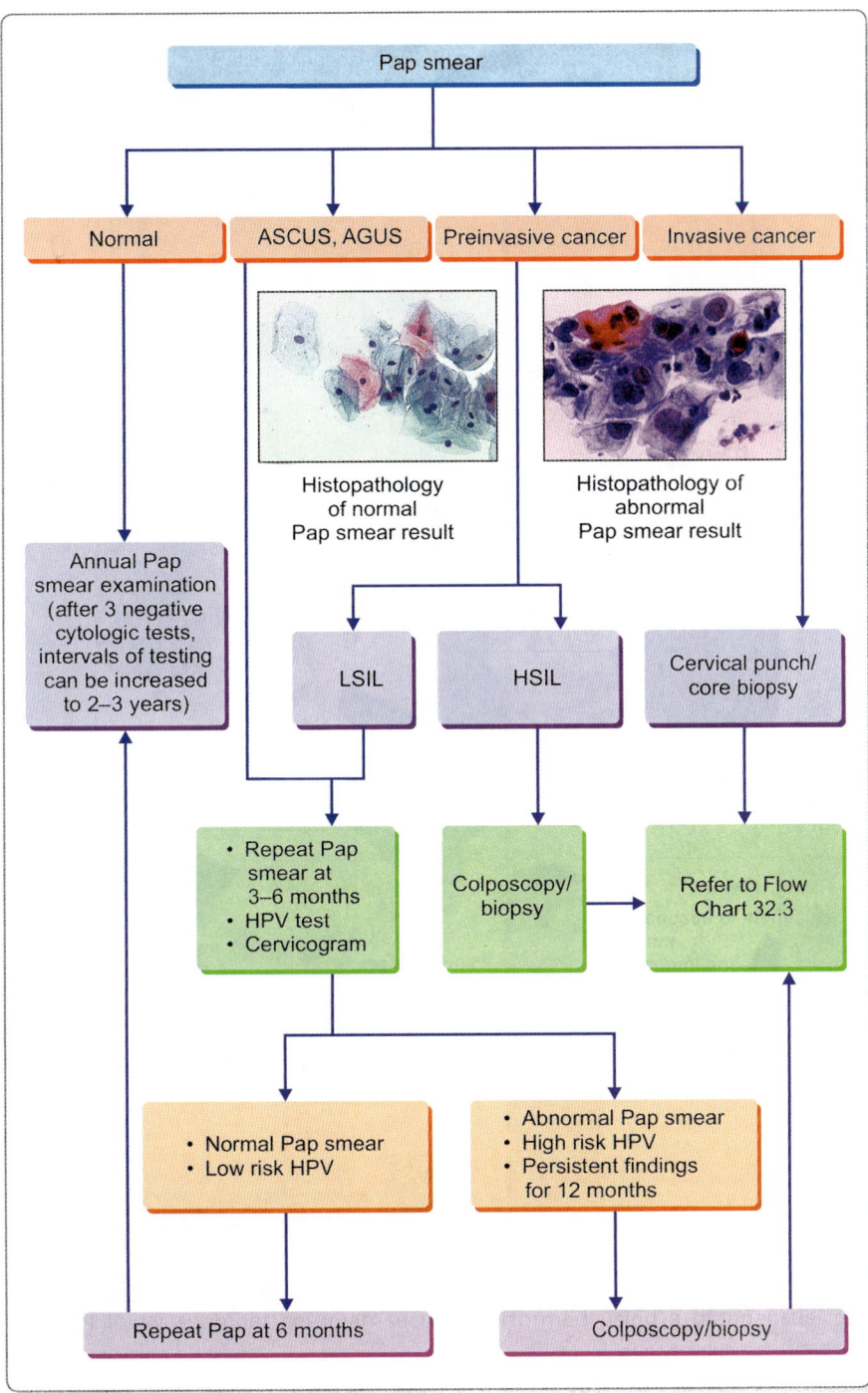

Flow Chart 32.2 Management of abnormal pap smears

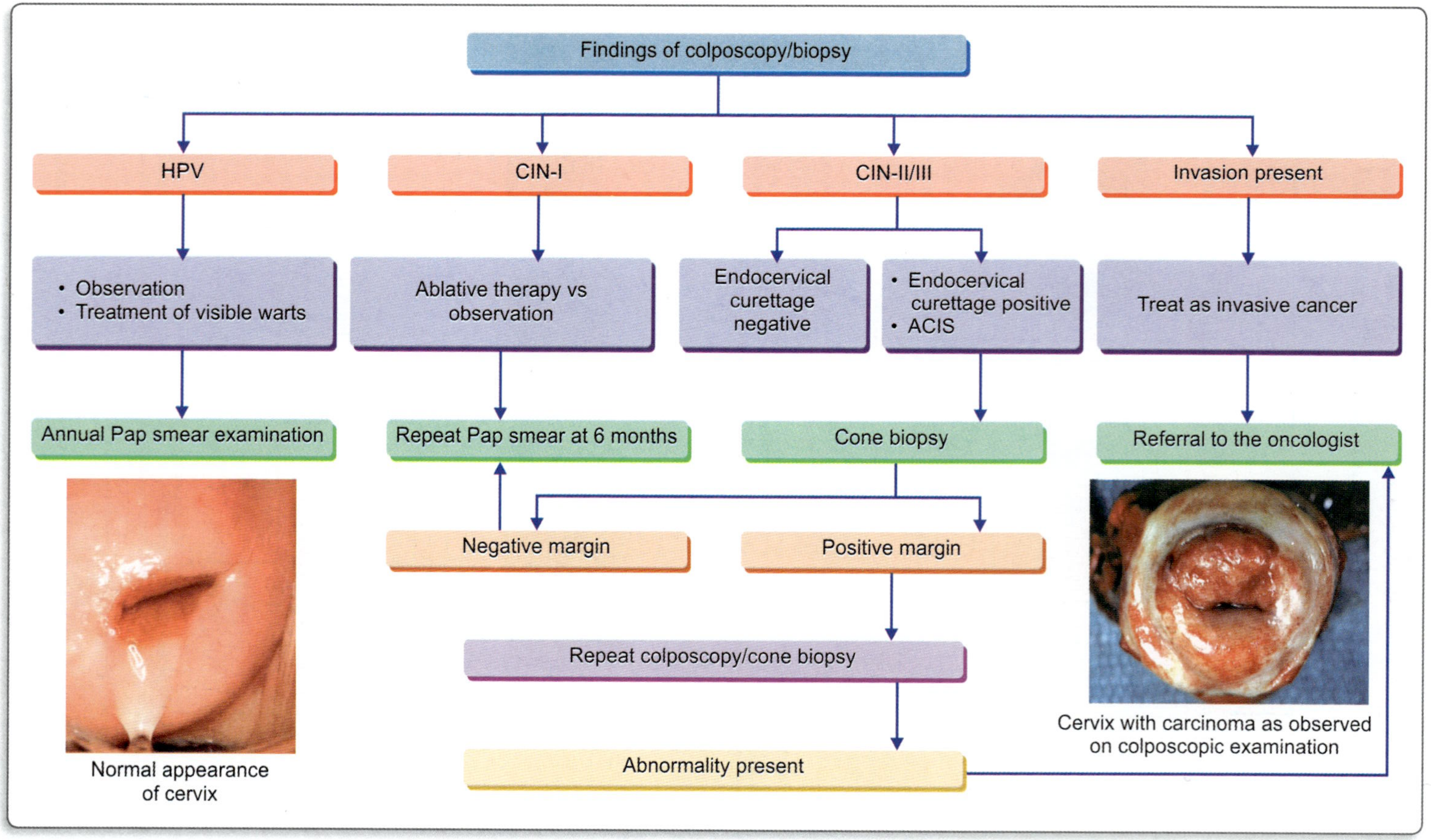

Section 10 ❖ Malignancies of the Genital Tract

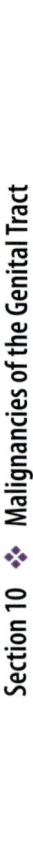

Flow Chart 32.3 Management of abnormal findings on colposcopy

33. Ovarian Neoplasms

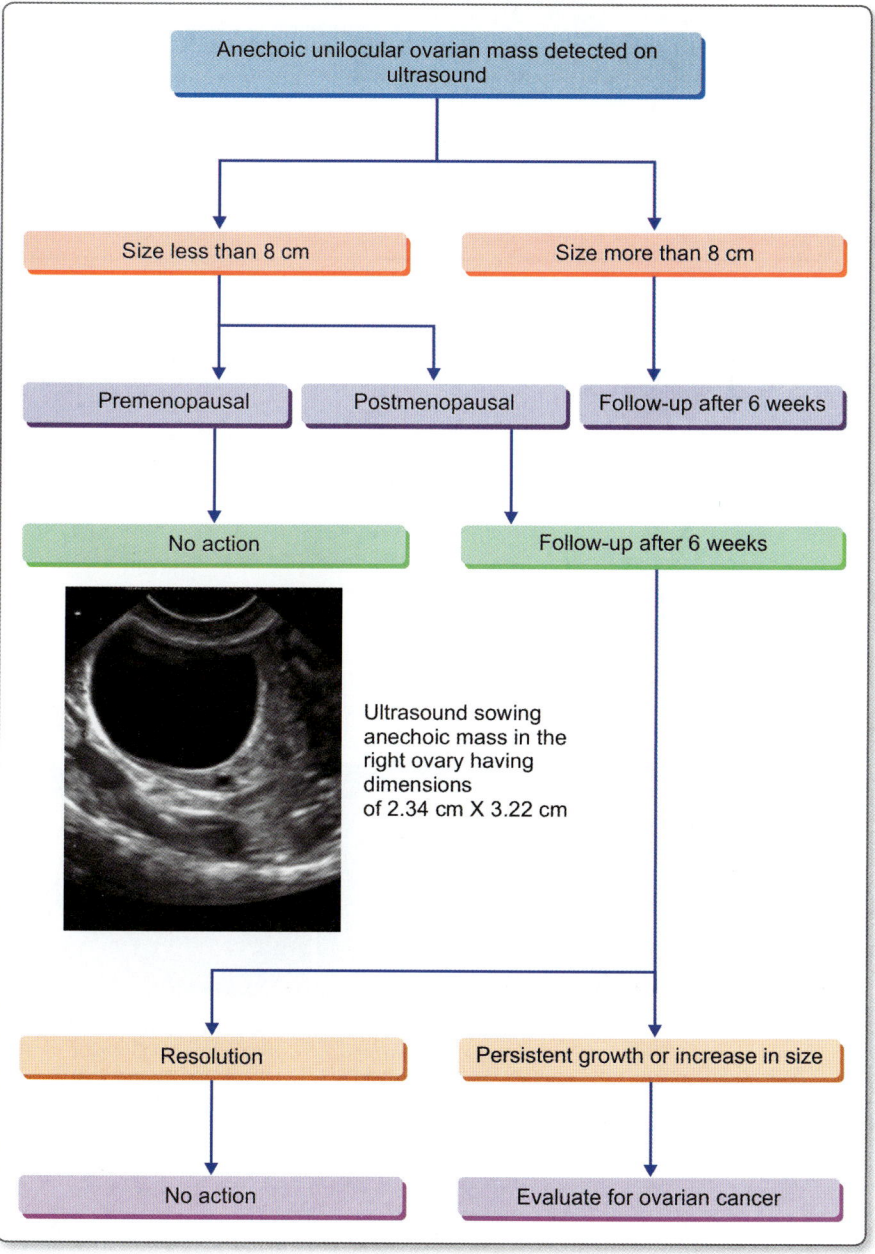

Flow Chart 33.1 Evaluation of anechoic adnexal mass

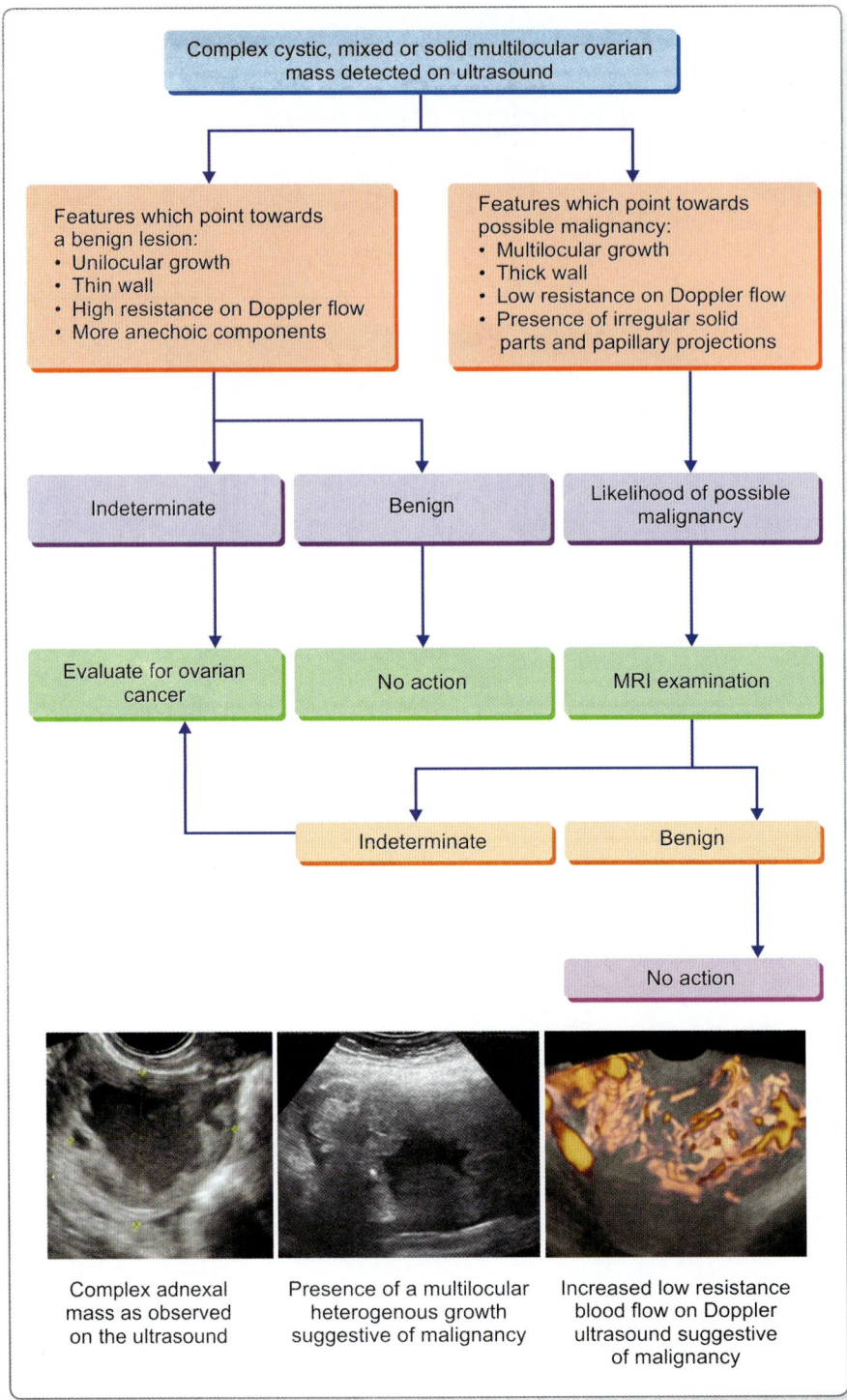

Flow Chart 33.2 Evaluation of complex cystic or solid adnexal mass

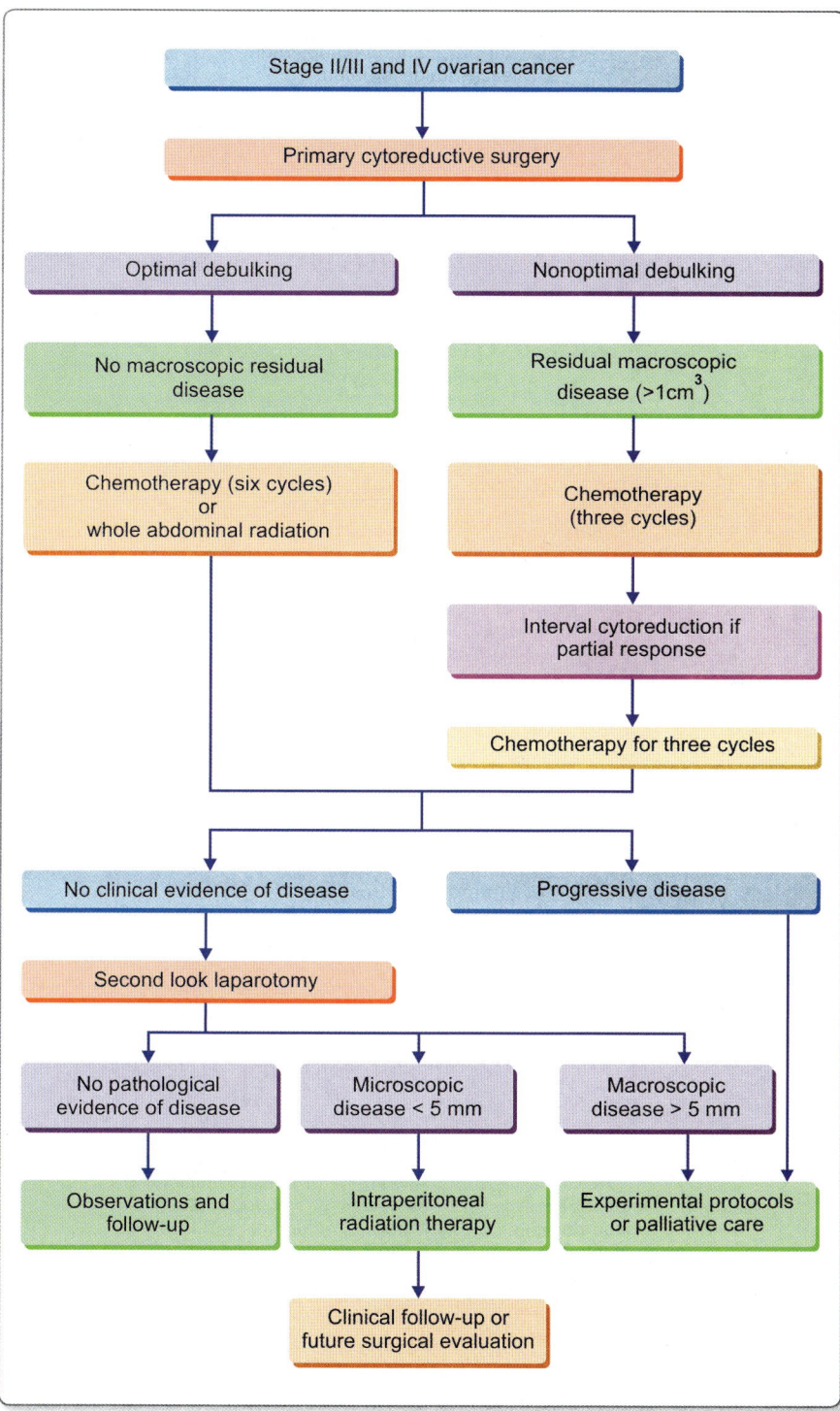

Flow Chart 33.3 Treatment plan for advanced stage epithelial ovarian cancer

GYNECOLOGY

Section 11 — Pain

- **Chapter 34**   Pelvic Pain
- **Chapter 35**   Ectopic Pregnancy
- **Chapter 36**   Dysmenorrhea

34. Pelvic Pain

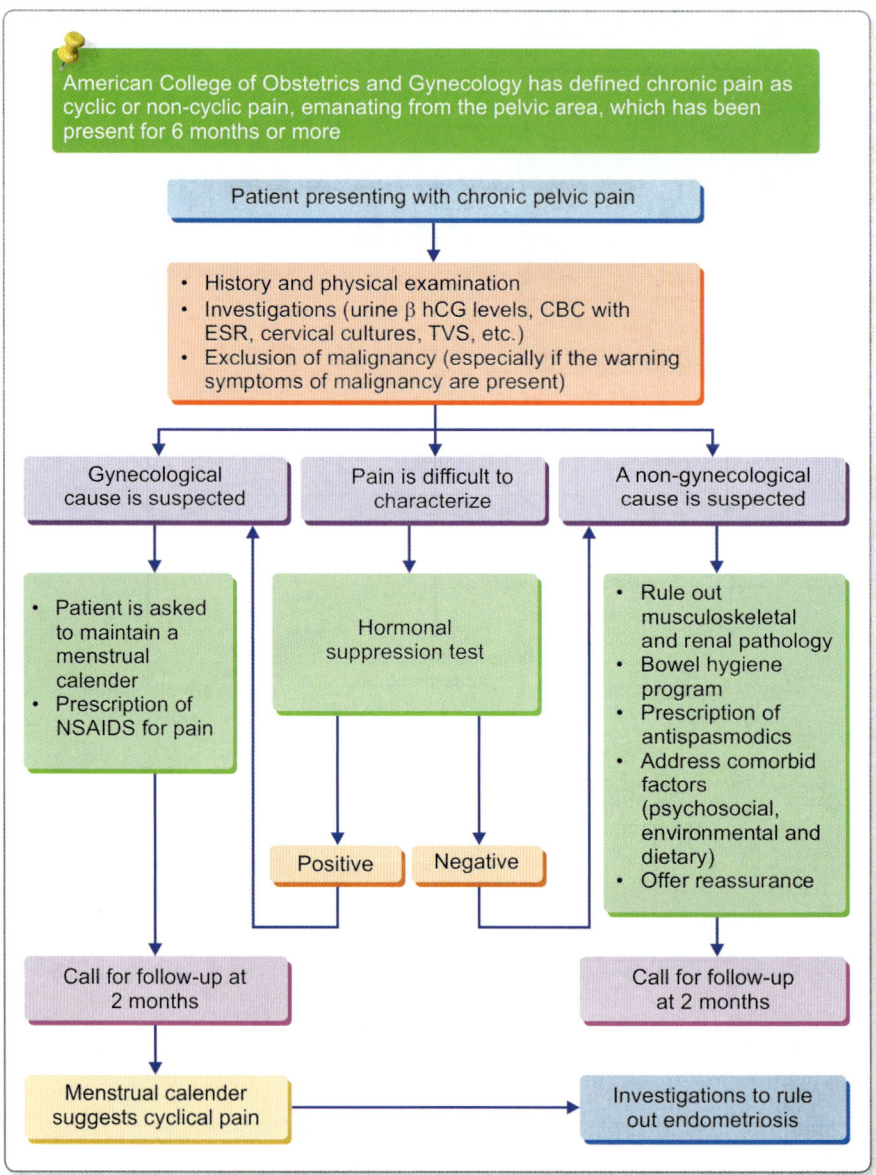

Flow Chart 34.1 Management of chronic pelvic pain in women

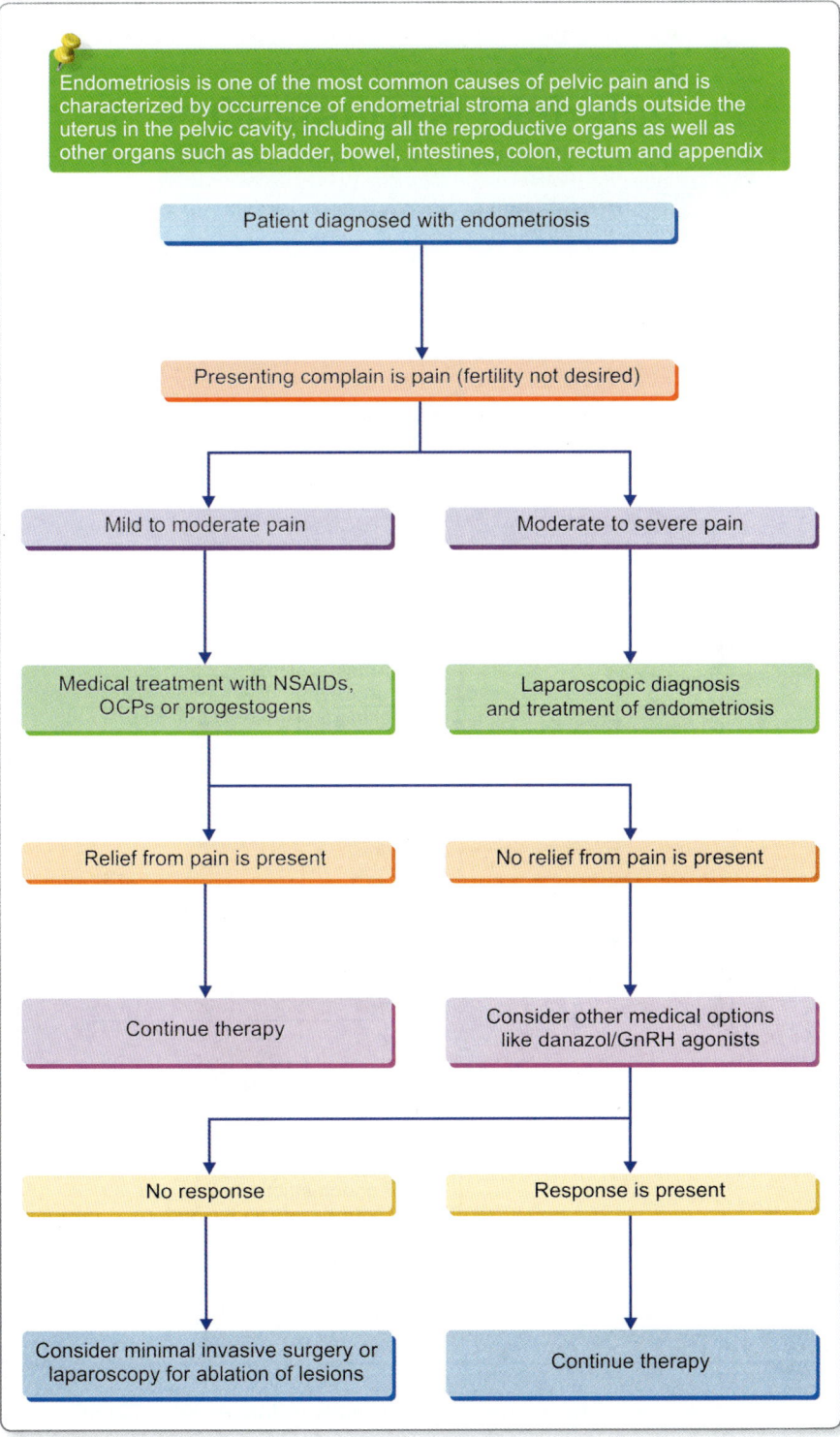

Flow Chart 34.2 Treatment of patients with endometriosis when the presenting complaint is pain

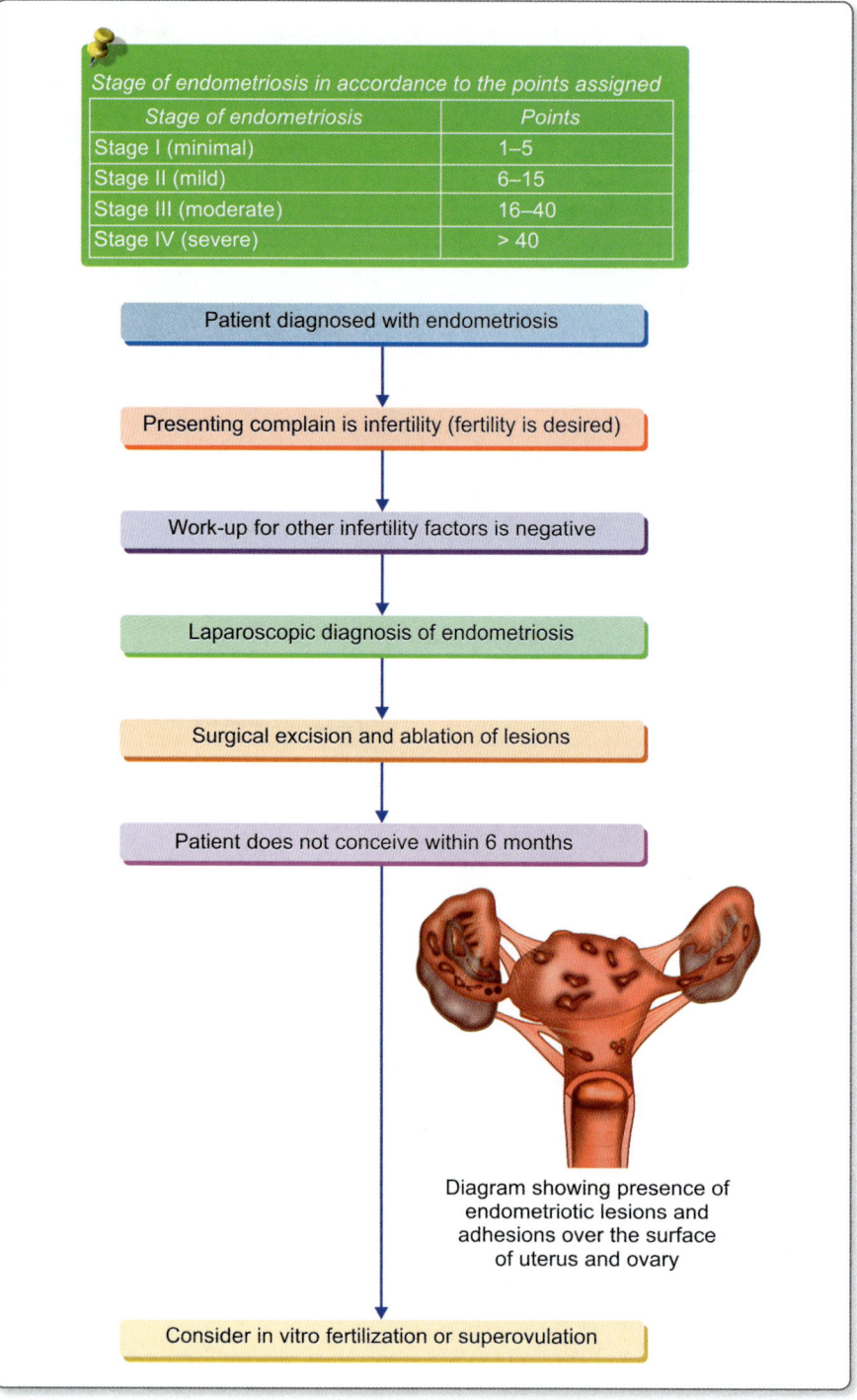

Flow Chart 34.3 Treatment of patients with endometriosis when the presenting complaint is infertility

Revised American Fertility Society classification of endometriosis (1996)

PERITONEUM			
Endometriosis	< 1 cm	1–3 cm	> 3 cm
Superficial	1	2	4
Deep	2	4	6

OVARY			
Right superficial	1	2	4
Right deep	4	16	20
Left superficial	1	2	4
Left deep	4	16	20

POSTERIOR CUL-DE-SAC OBLITERATION	
Partial	Complete
4	40

OVARY			
Adhesions	< 1/3 enclosure	1/3–2/3 enclosure	> 2/3 enclosure3
Right filmy	1	2	4
Right dense	4	8	16
Left filmy	1	2	4
Left dense	4	8	16

TUBE			
Right filmy	1	2	4
Right dense	4*	8*	16
Left filmy	1	2	4
Left dense	4*	8*	16

*If the fimbriated end of the fallopian tube is completely enclosed, the point assignment is changed to 16

Revised American Society for Reproductive Medicne classification of endometriosis

Source: Revised American Society for Reproductive Medicne classification of endometriosis: 1996. Fertil Steril. 1997;67:817–21.

35 Ectopic Pregnancy

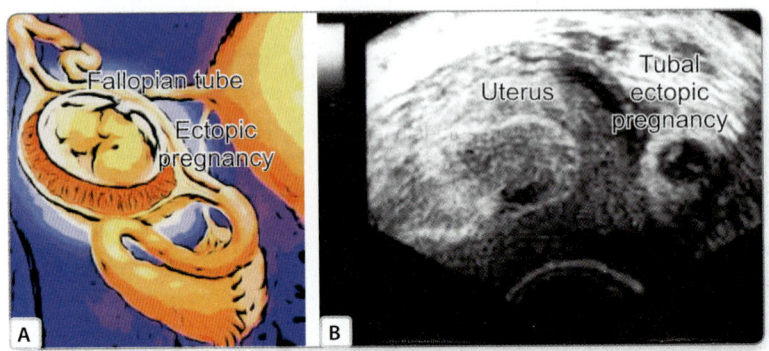

(A) Artist's interpretation of ectopic pregnancy, implying that the pregnancy occurs outside the uterine cavity; (B) Ultrasound showing ectopic pregnancy in the left tube

The criteria for TVS diagnosis of ectopic pregnancy	
Type	TVS finding
Type 1A	Well-defined tubal ring displaying fetal heart
Type 1B	Well-defined tubal ring displaying no fetal heart
Type 2	Ill-defined tubal mass
Type 3	Free pelvic fluid, empty uterus, displaying no adnexal mass

Criteria for the diagnosis of ectopic pregnancy through transvaginal ultrasound examination

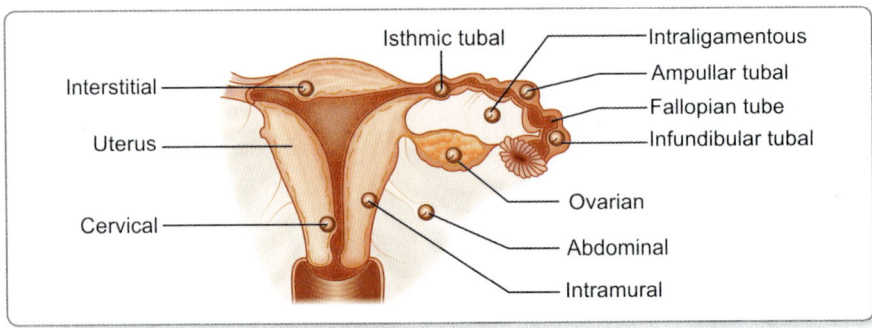

Common sites for the occurence of ectopic pregnancy

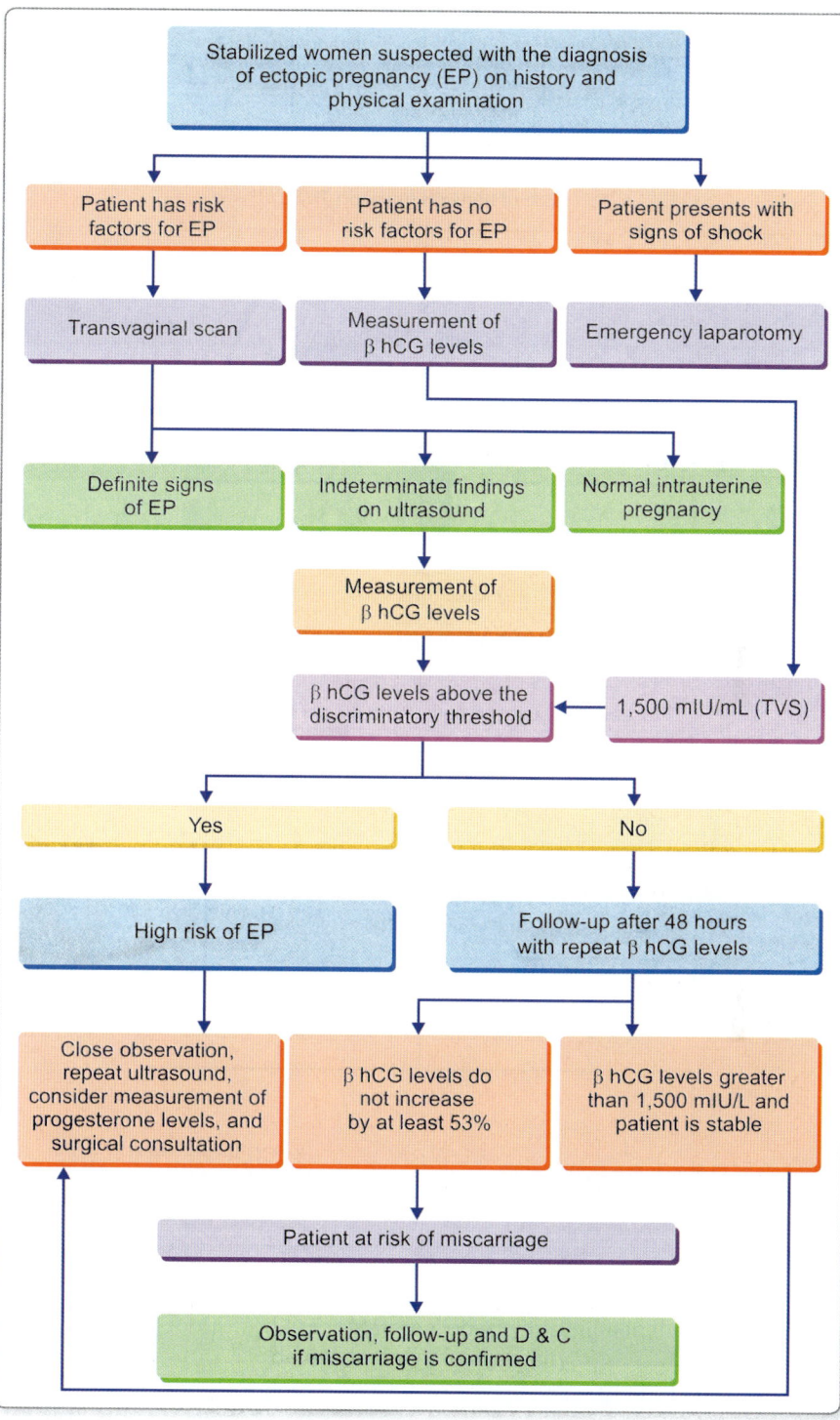

Flow Chart 35.1 Management of stable patients with suspected diagnosis of ectopic pregnancy

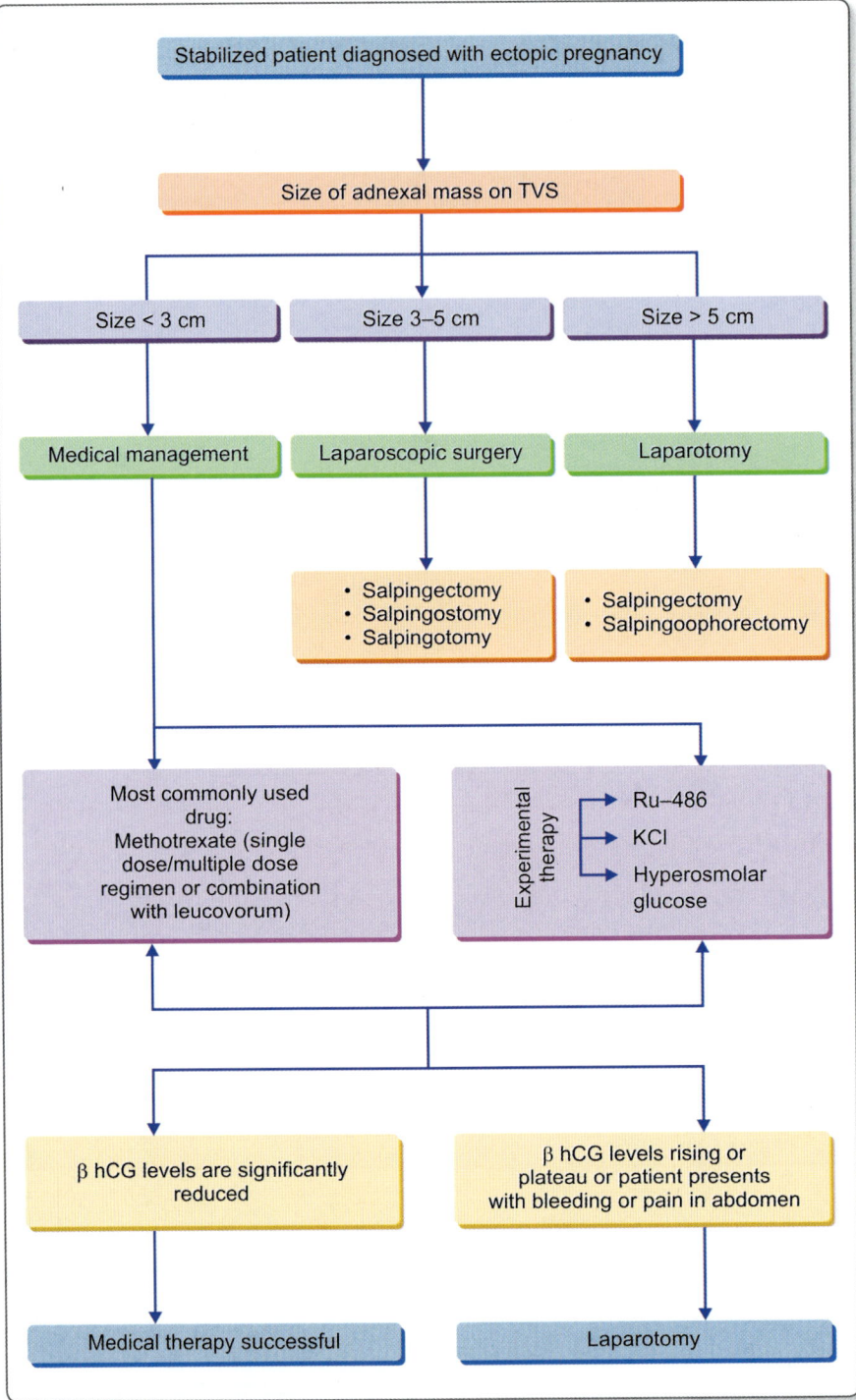

Flow Chart 35.2 Treatment plan for patients with suspected diagnosis of ectopic pregnancy

36 Dysmenorrhea

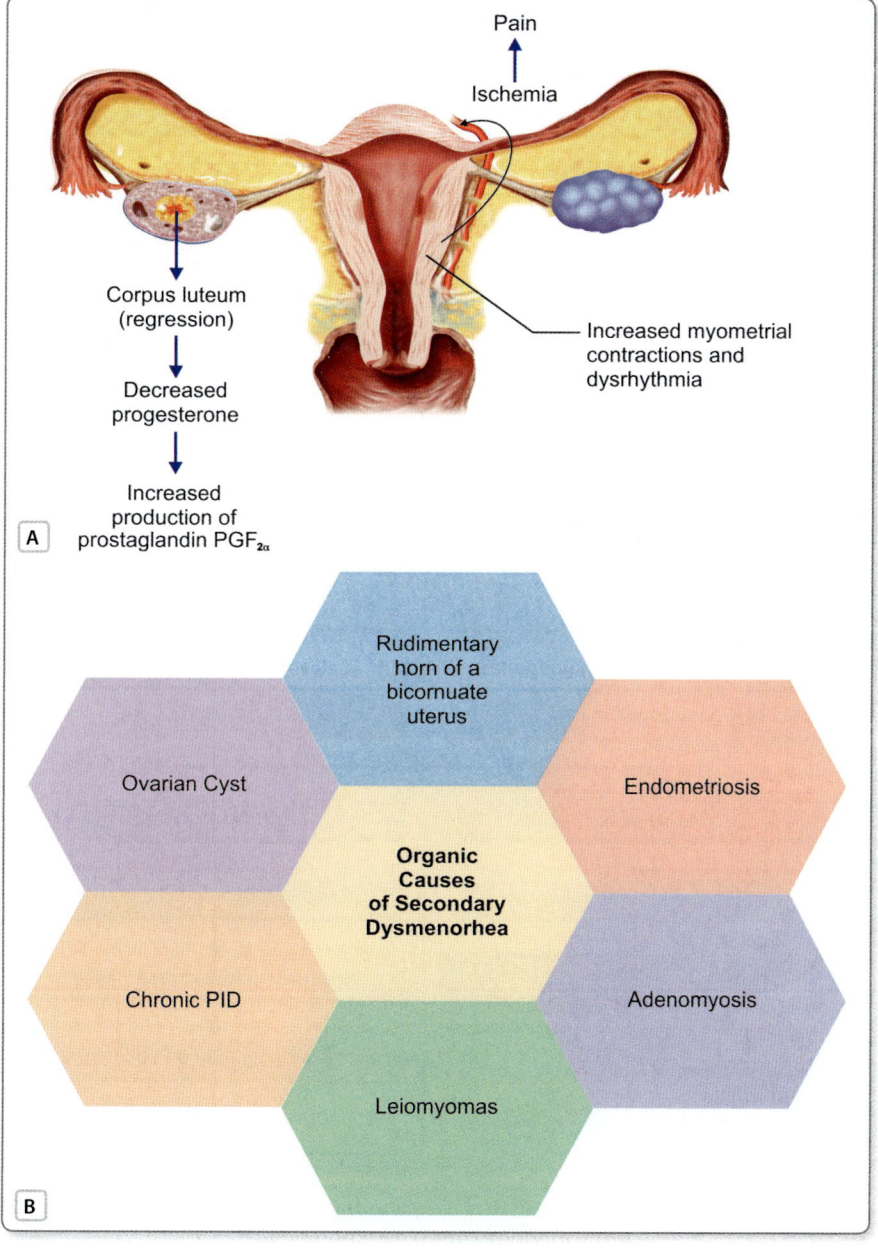

A. Mechanism of primary dysmenorrhea; B. Causes of secondary dymenorrhea

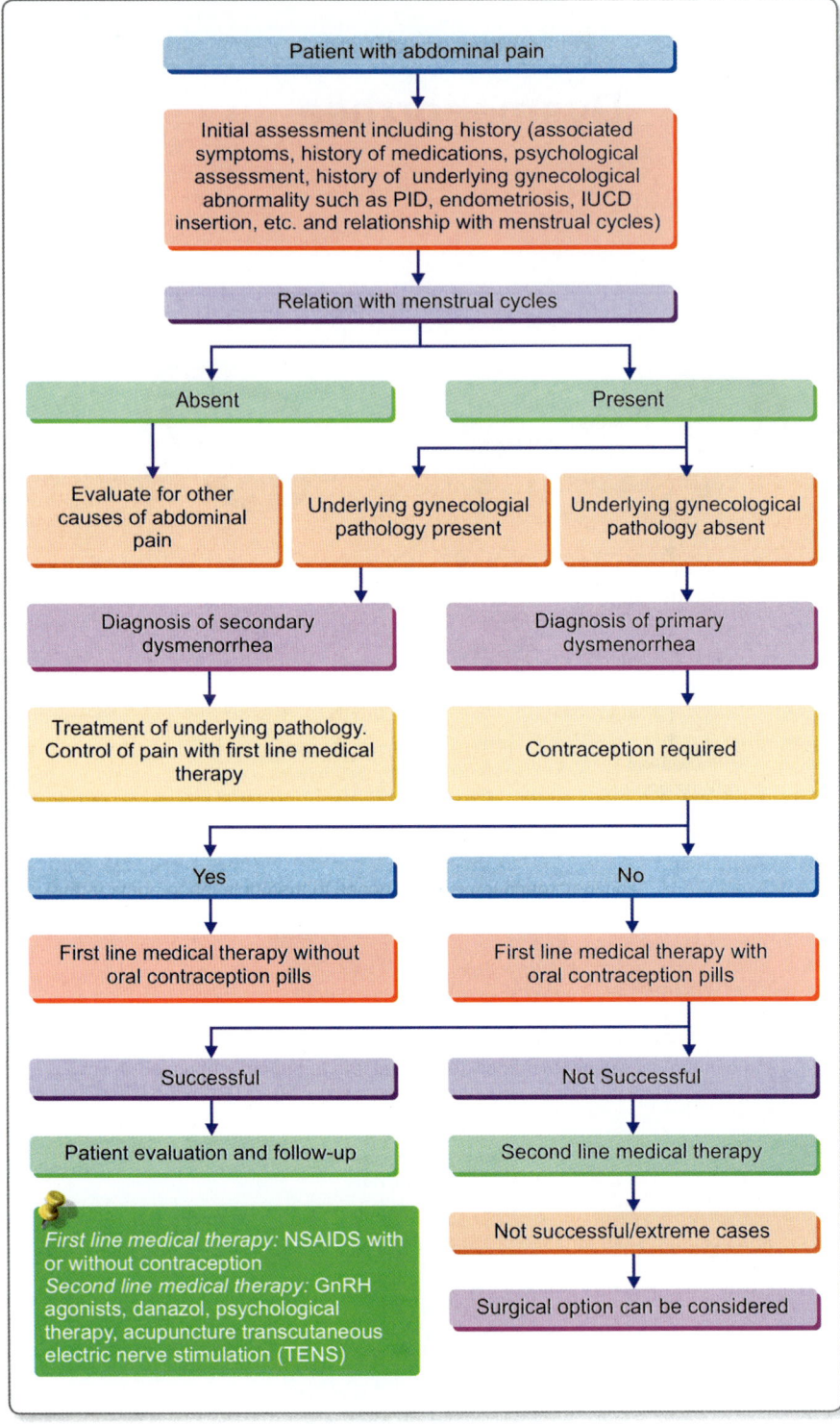

Flow Chart 36.1 Management of cases of dysmenorrhea

GYNECOLOGY

Section 12

Abnormalities in Conception

- **Chapter 37** Infertility
- **Chapter 38** Amenorrhea
- **Chapter 39** Polycystic Ovarian Syndrome
- **Chapter 40** Hirsutism

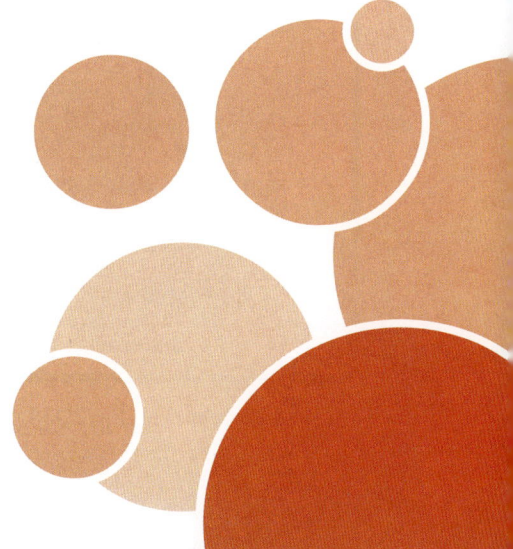

37 Infertility

Definition
Infertility is defined as the inability to conceive even after trying with unprotected intercourse for a period of 1 year for couples in whom the woman is under 35 years and 6 months of trying for couples in which the woman is over 35 years of age

Definition of infertility

Causes of infertility

Causes of infertility	Percentage of cases
Female causes	30%
Male causes	30%
Both male and female partner	30%
Unexplained causes	10%

Various causes of infertility

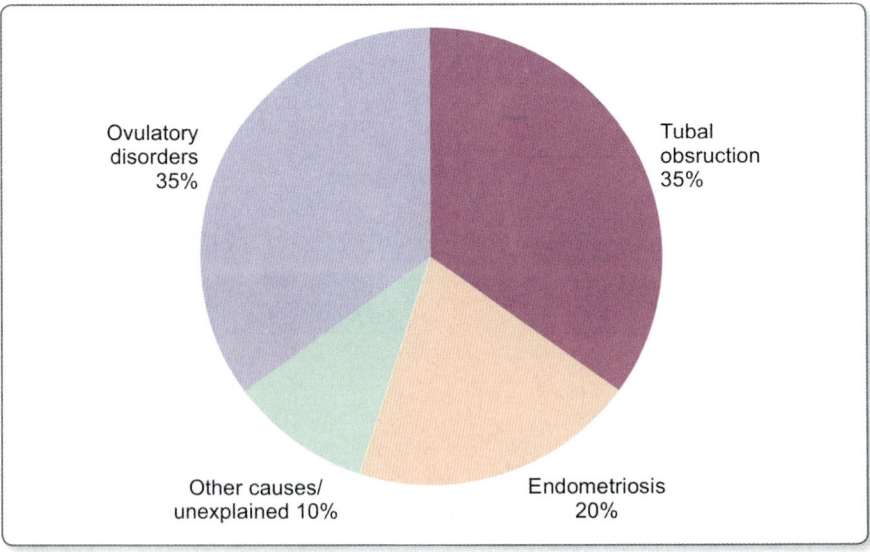

Female causes of infertility

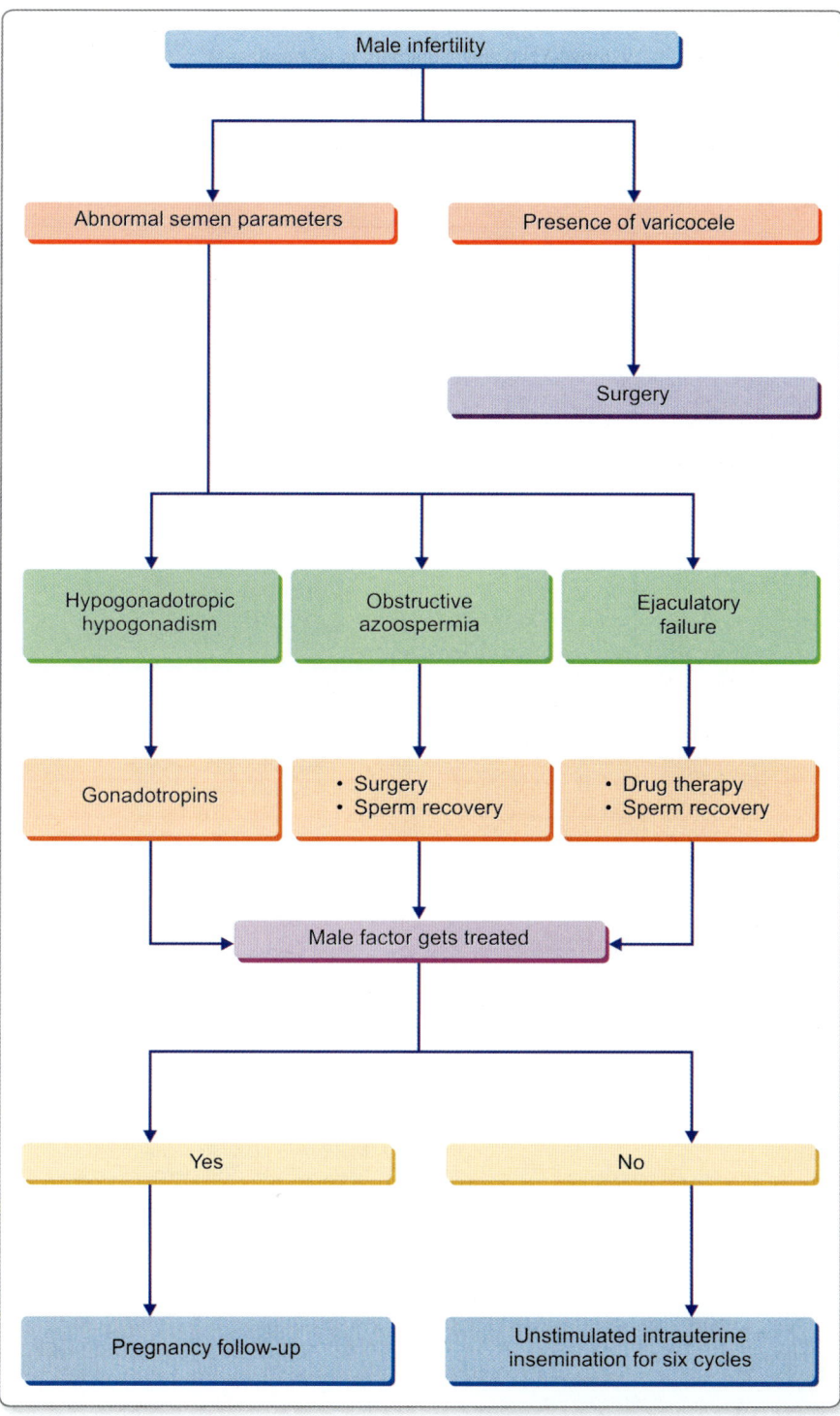

Flow Chart 37.1 Treatment of male infertility

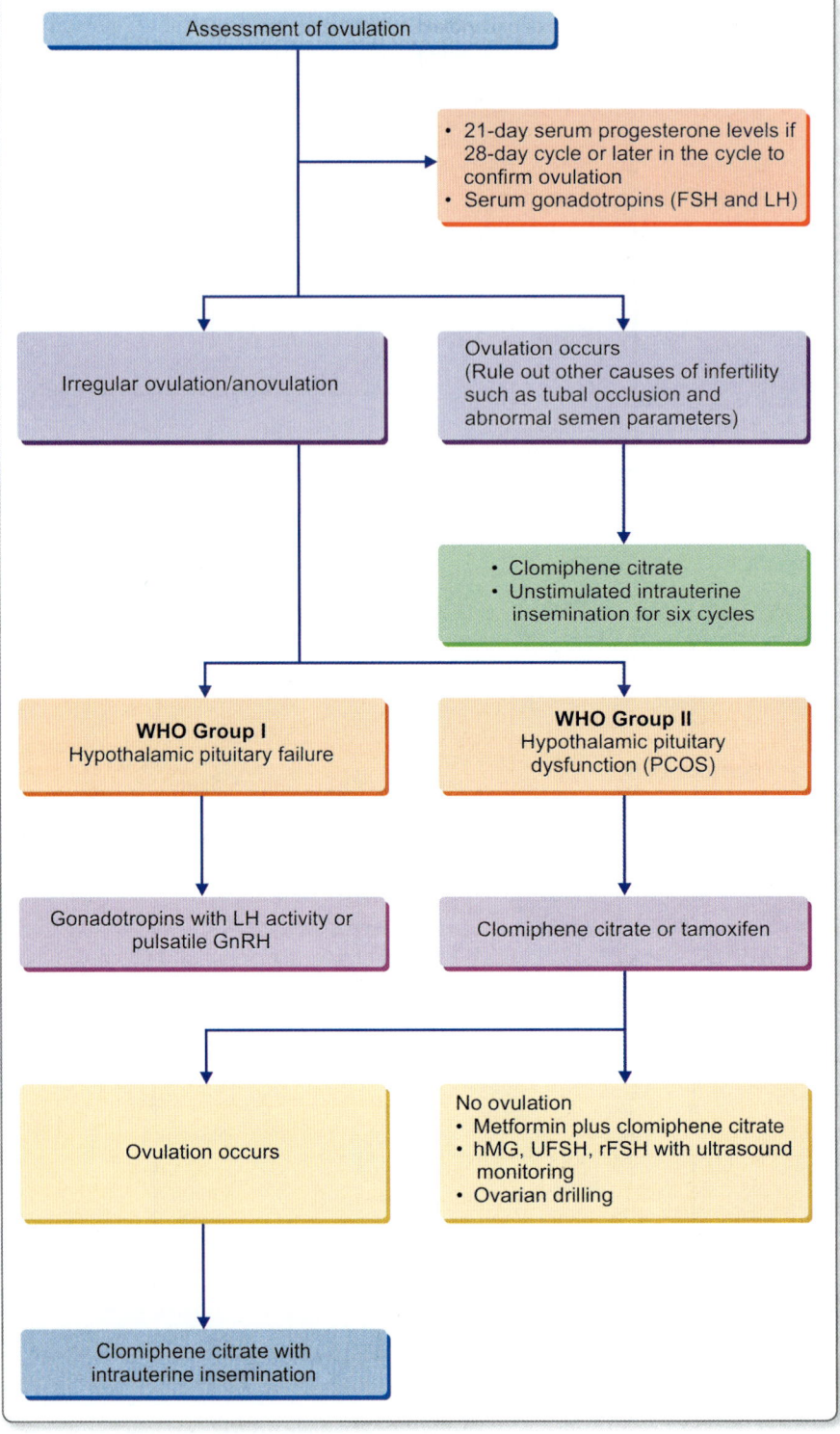

Flow Chart 37.2 Treatment of infertility due to ovarian factors

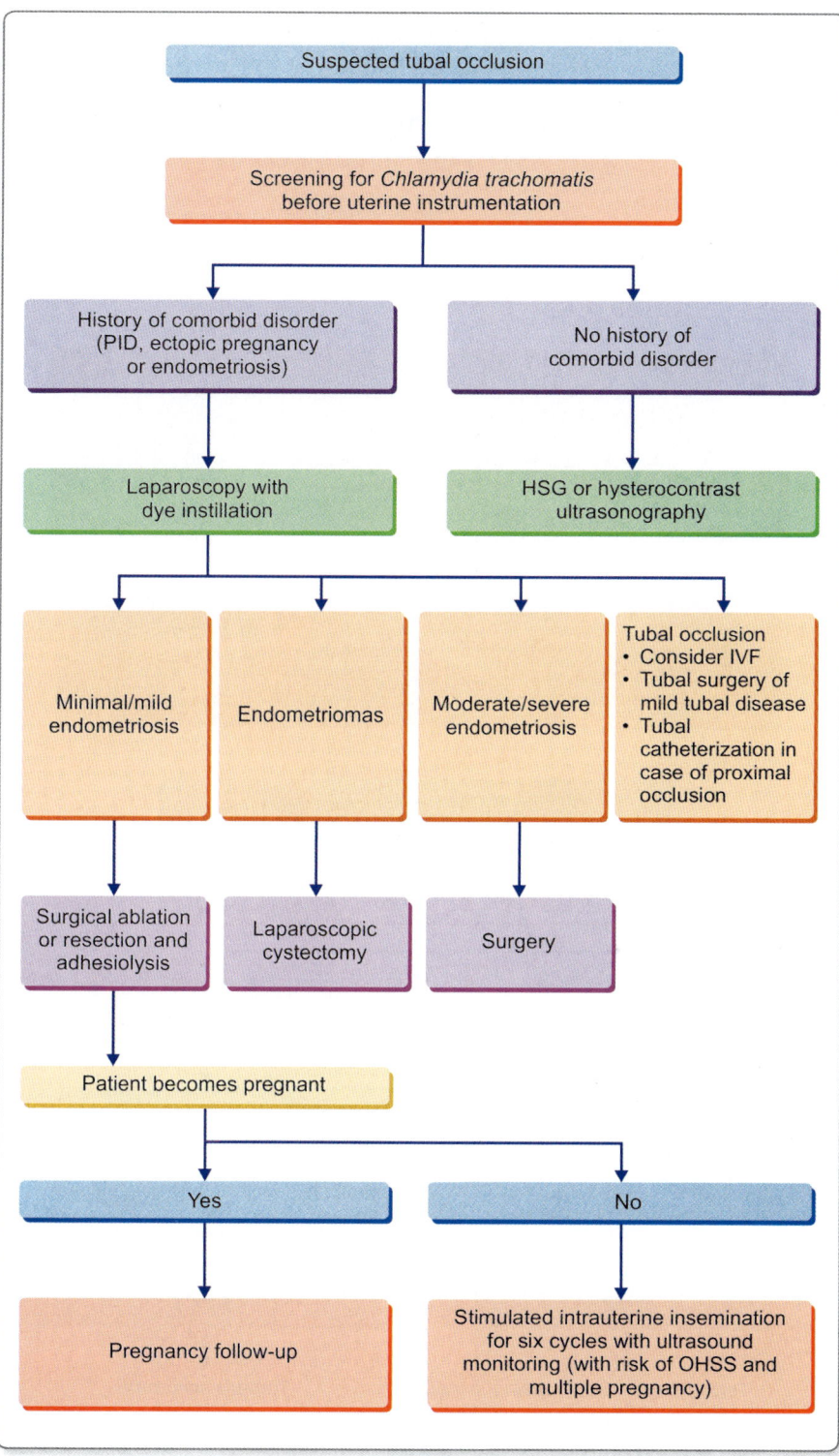

Flow Chart 37.3 Treatment of tubal disease

38 Amenorrhea

Amenorrhea implies absence of menstrual periods and can be of two types: primary and secondary. Primary amenorrhea is absence of menstrual cycles in a woman who had never experienced menstrual cycles before. Secondary amenorrhea, on the other hand, is defined as the cessation of menstruation in a woman who had been previously experiencing menstrual bleeding. This cessation must last for at least 6 months or for at least 3 of the previous 3-cycle intervals

Primary amenorrhea can be defined as follows:
- Absence of menses by age of 14 years with the absence of growth or development of secondary sexual characteristics
- Or absence of menses by the age of 16 years with normal development of secondary sexual characteristics

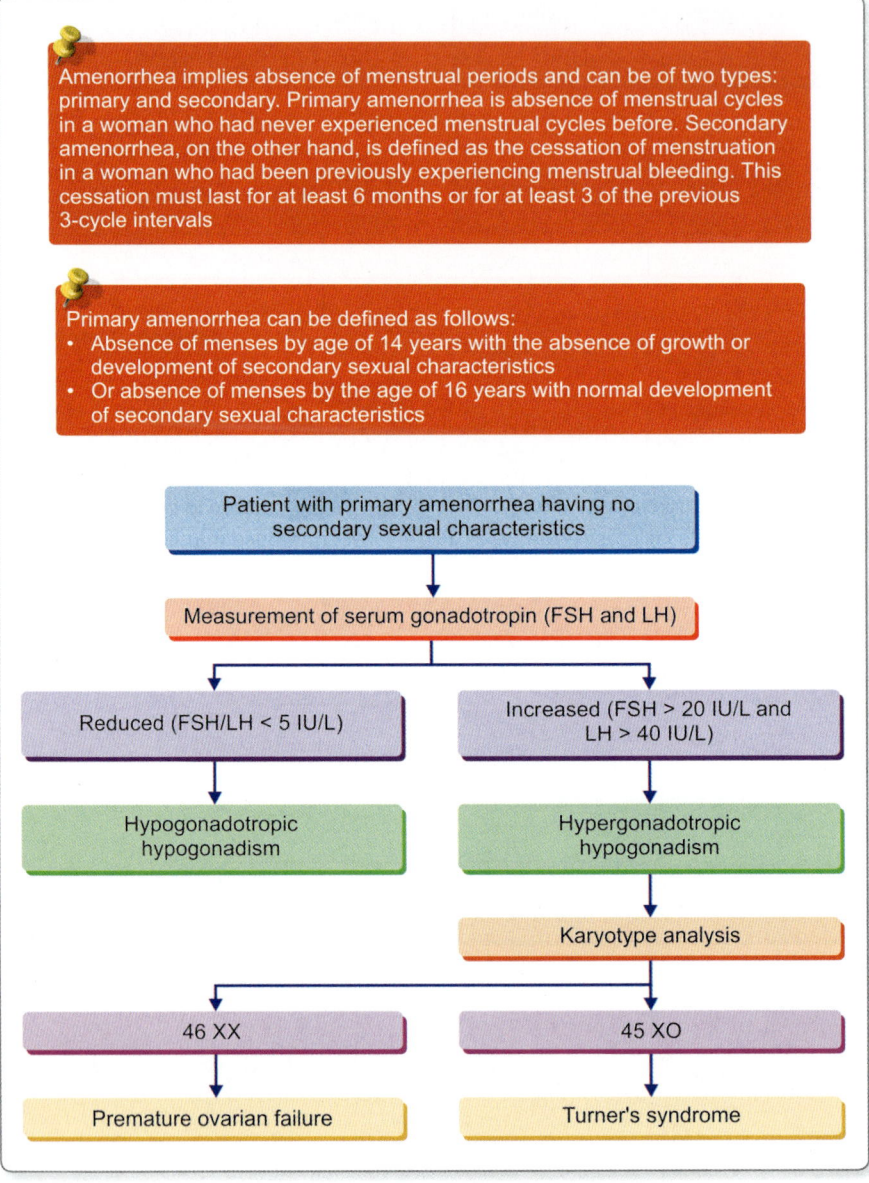

Flow Chart 38.1 Evaluation of a patient with primary amenorrhea having no secondary sexual characteristics

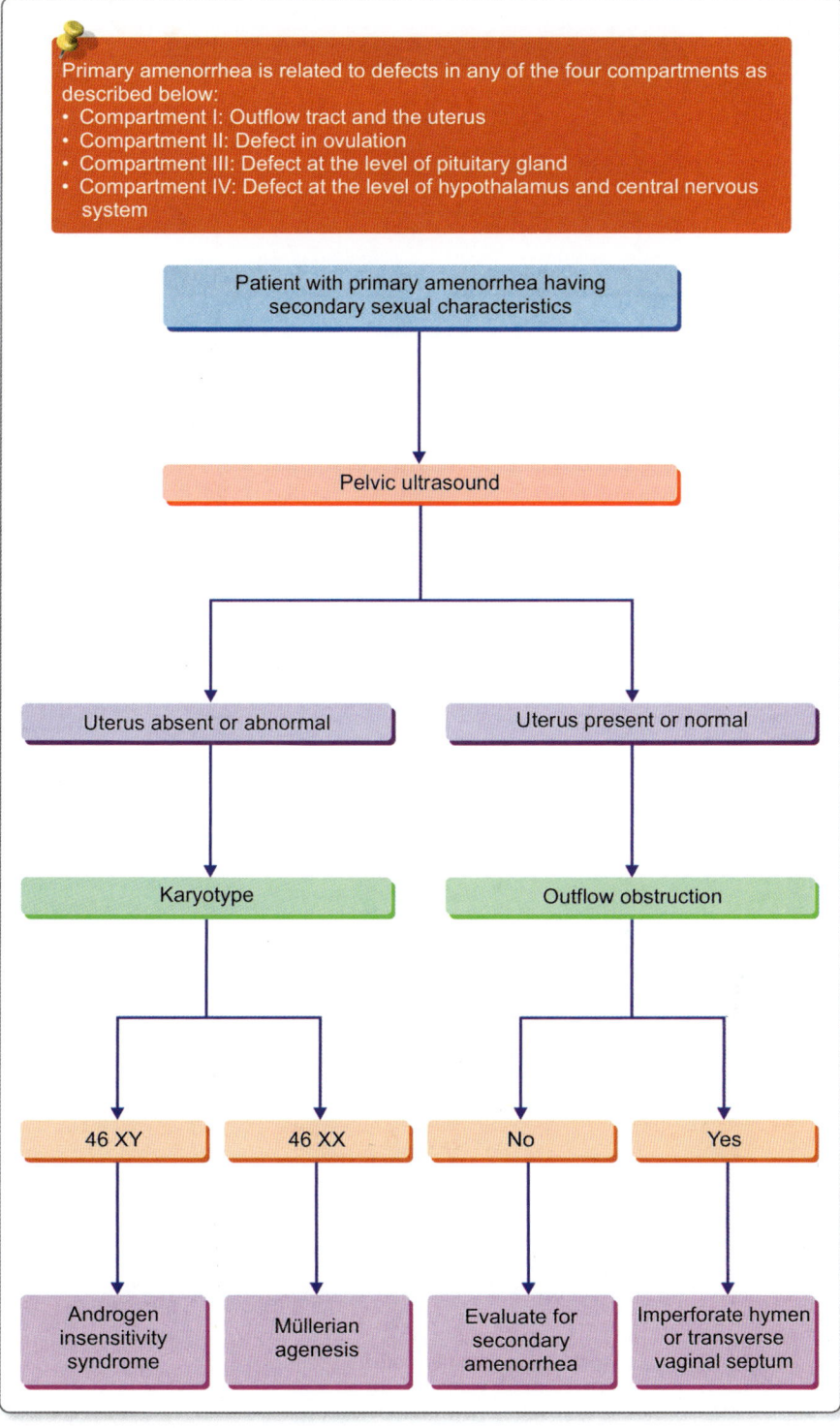

Flow Chart 38.2 Evaluation of a patient with primary amenorrhea having secondary sexual characteristics

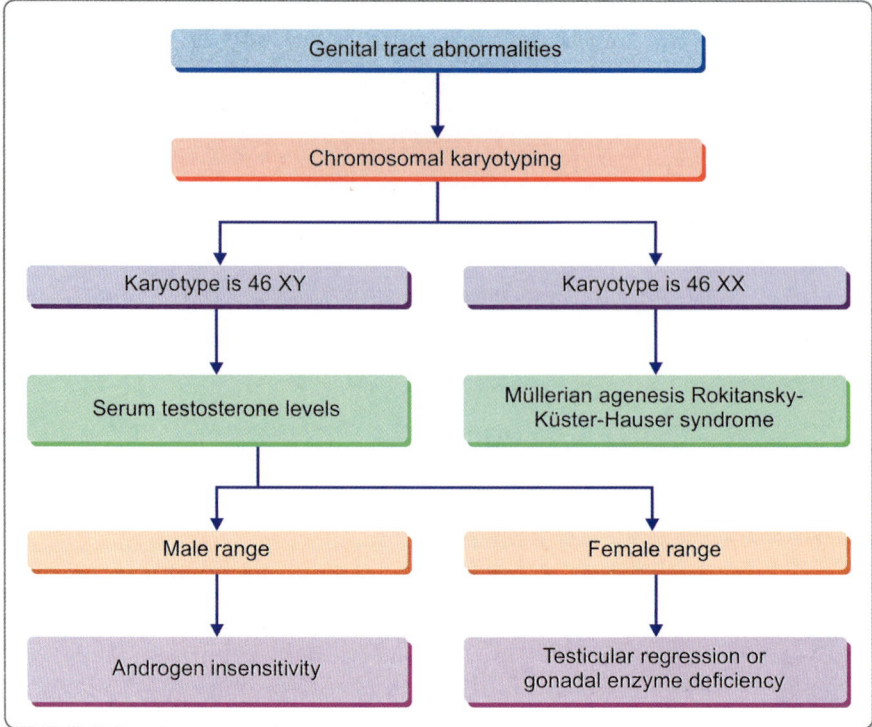

Flow Chart 38.3 Management protocol in case of genital tract abnormalities

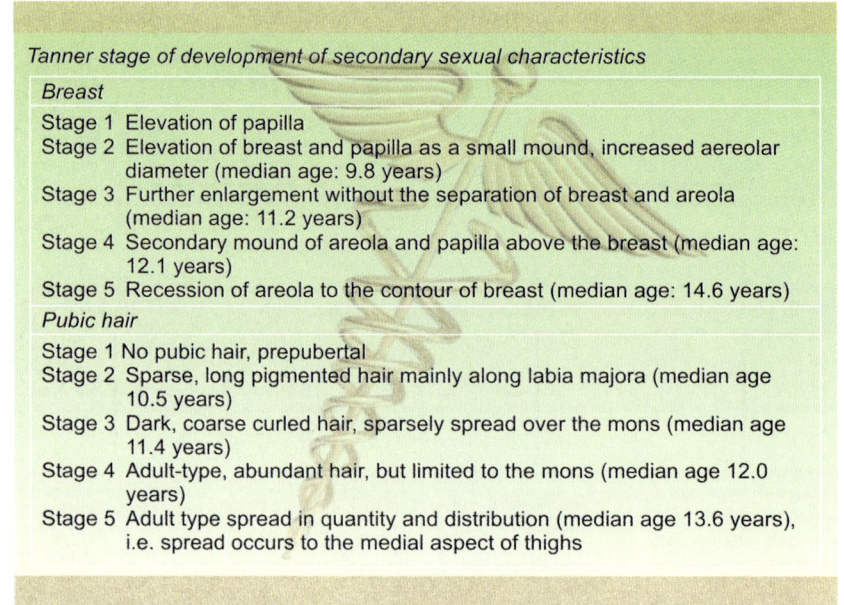

Tanner stage of development of secondary sexual characteristics

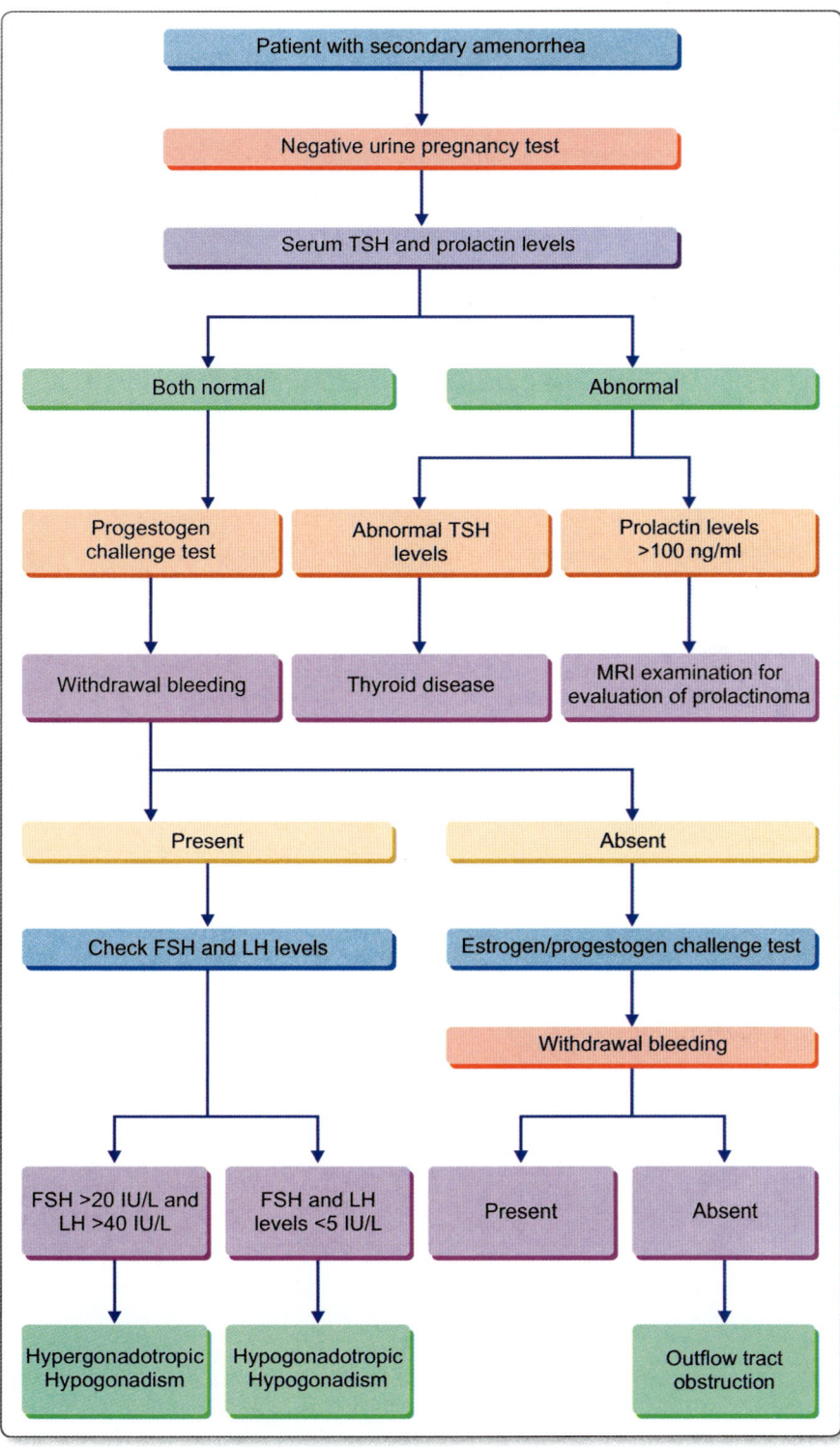

Flow Chart 38.4 Management plan in a patient with secondary amenorrhea having negative urine pregnancy test

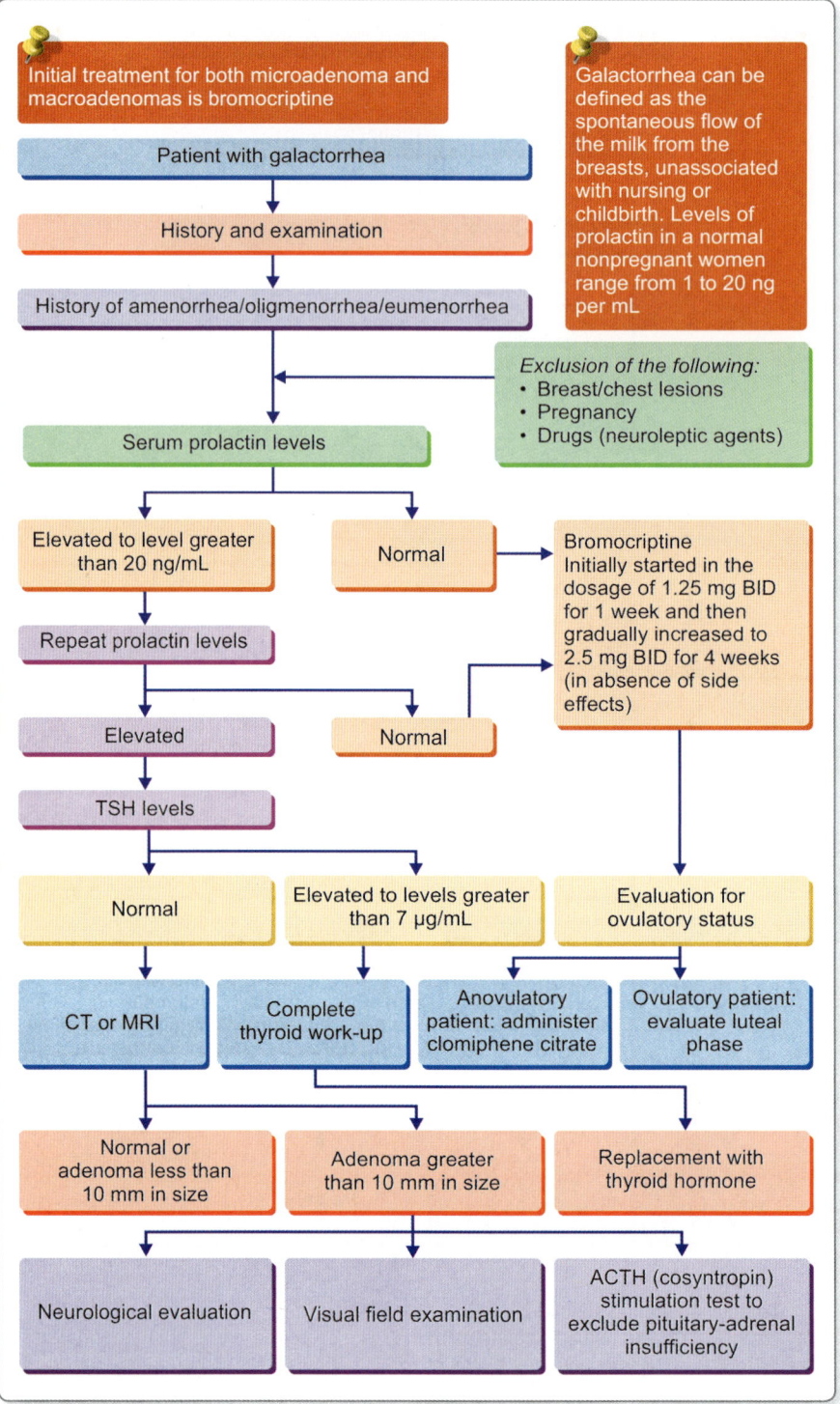

Flow Chart 38.5 Management of galactorrhea in an amenorrhic patient

39 Polycystic Ovarian Syndrome

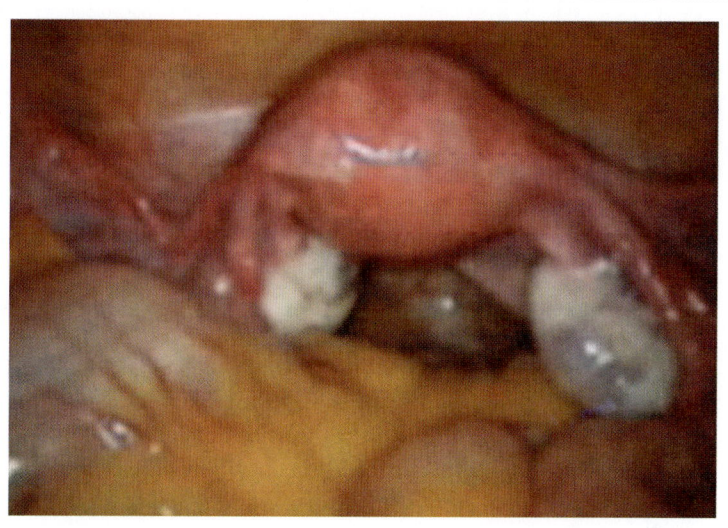

Bilateral polycystic ovaries as observed on laparoscopic examination

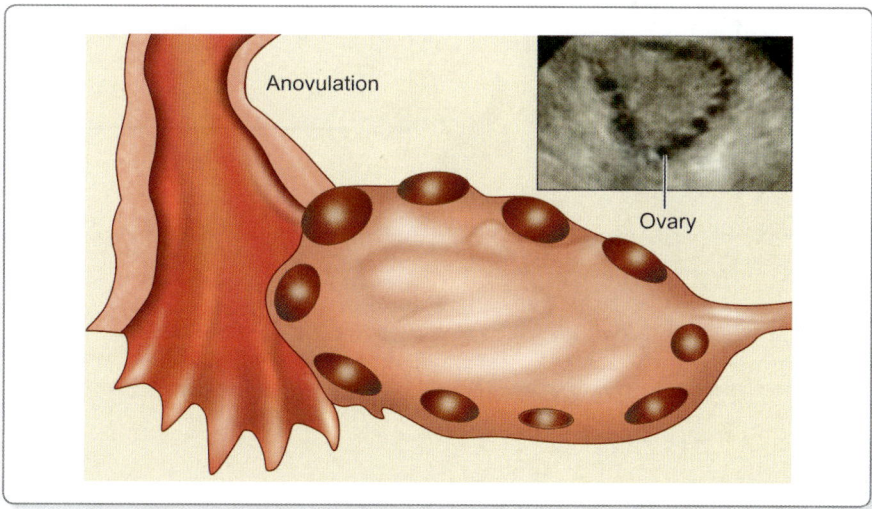

Comparison of polycystic ovary (gross and ultrasound appearance)

Section 12 ❖ Abnormalities in Conception

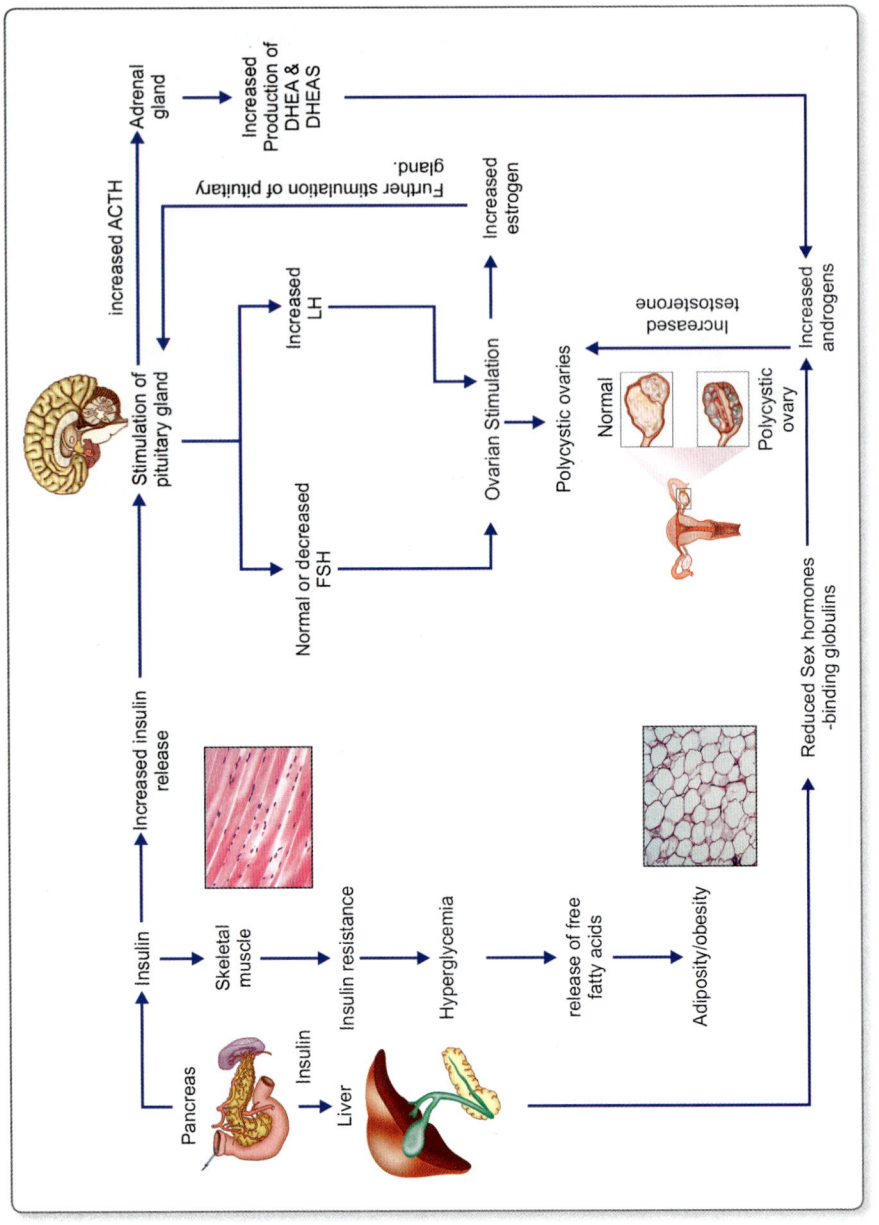

Flow Chart 39.1 Pathophysiology of PCOS

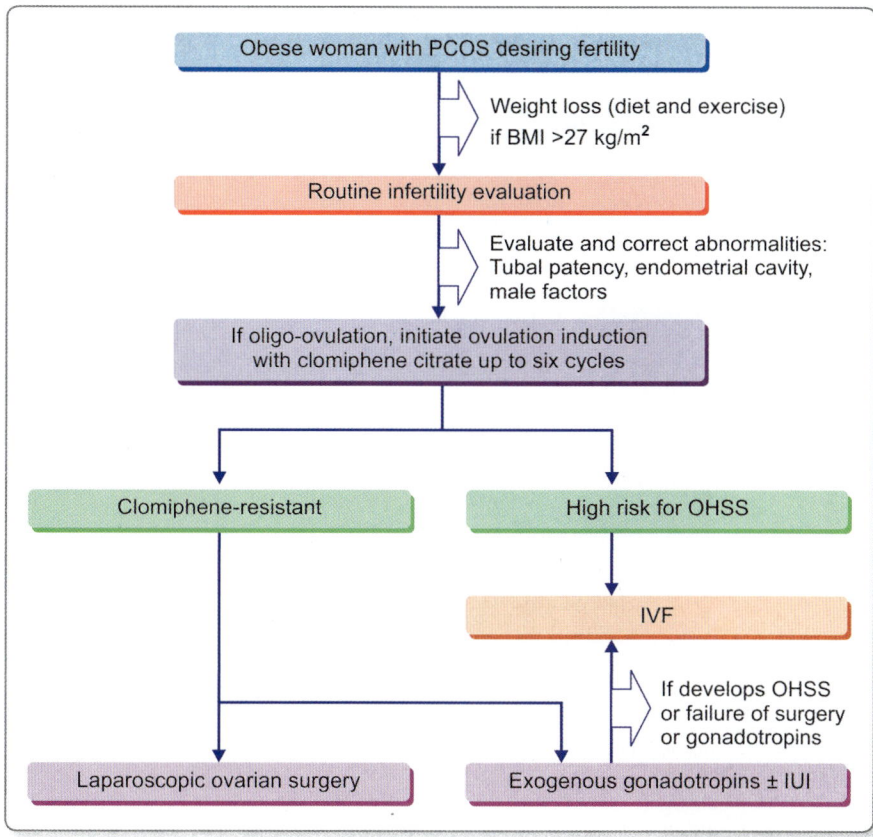

Flow Chart 39.2 Treatment of patients with PCOS desiring fertility

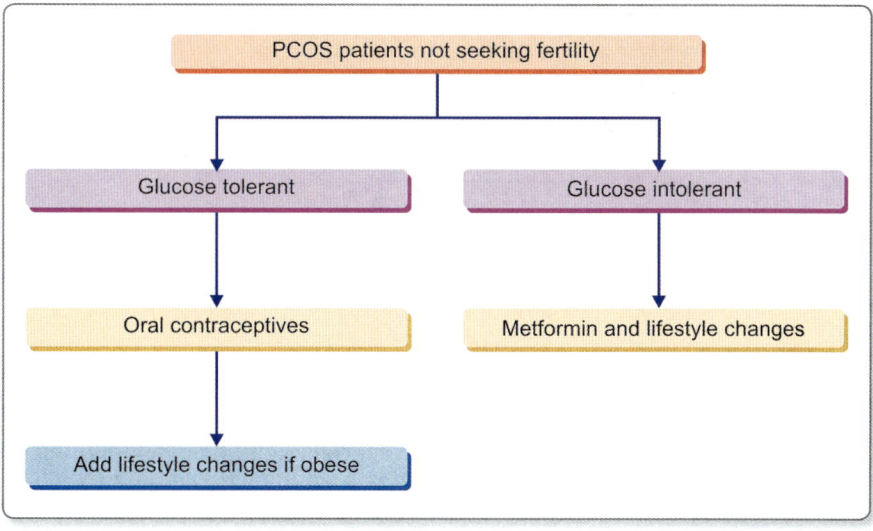

Flow Chart 39.3 Treatment of patients with PCOS not desiring fertility

40 Hirsutism

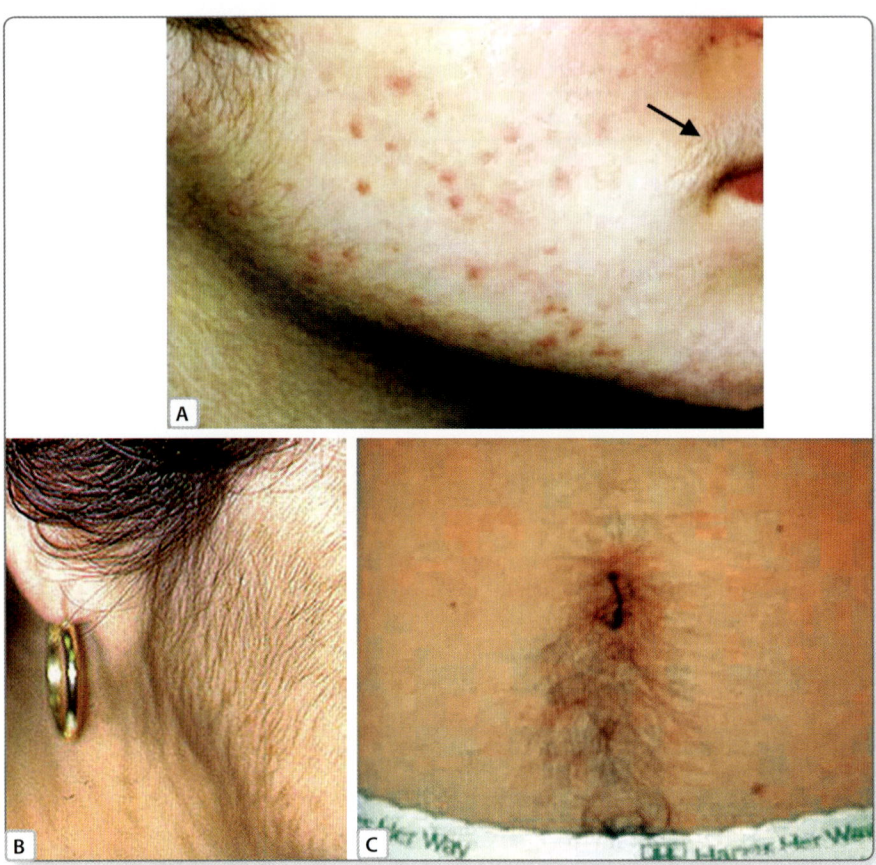

Hirsutism or excessive hair: (A) Over the upper lip; (B) Over the side burn area; (C) Abdominal hair

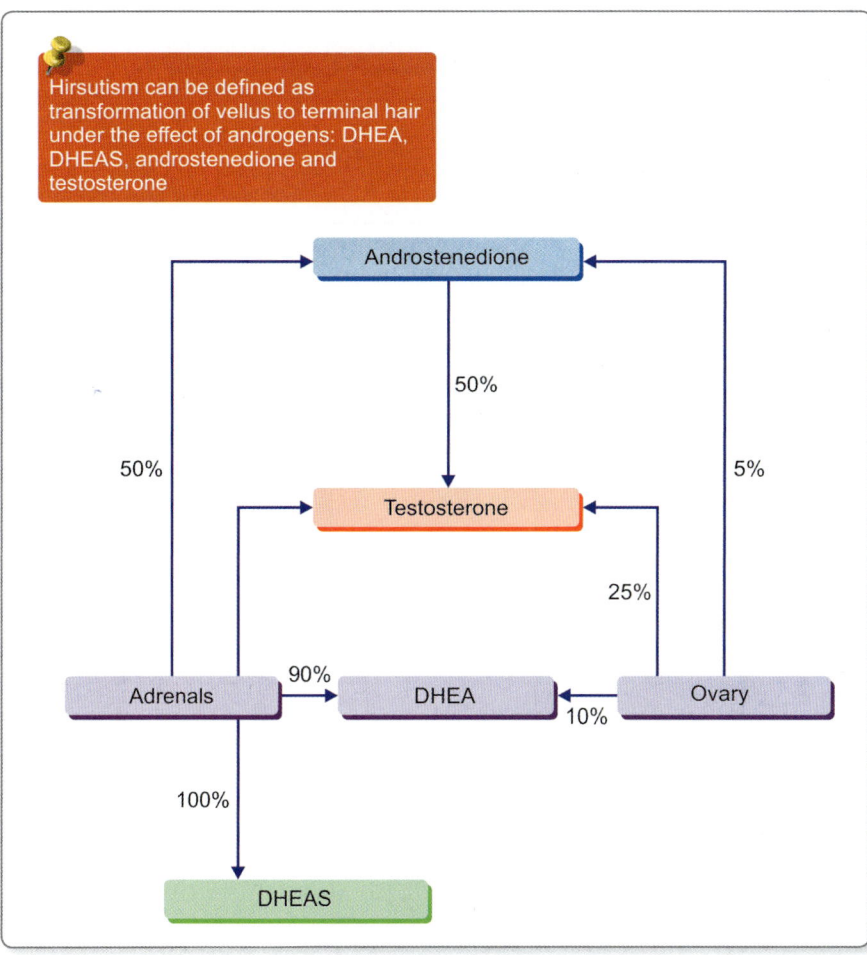

Flow Chart 40.1 Production of androgens from various sources

Causes of hirsutism	
Ovarian causes:	PCOS (90%), virilizing ovarian tumors, ovarian dysgenesis, etc.
Adrenal causes:	congenital adrenal hyperplasia
Peripheral causes:	idiopathic, insulin resistance
Drugs:	danazol, metoclopramide, methyldopa, testosterone, etc.

Various causes of hirsutism

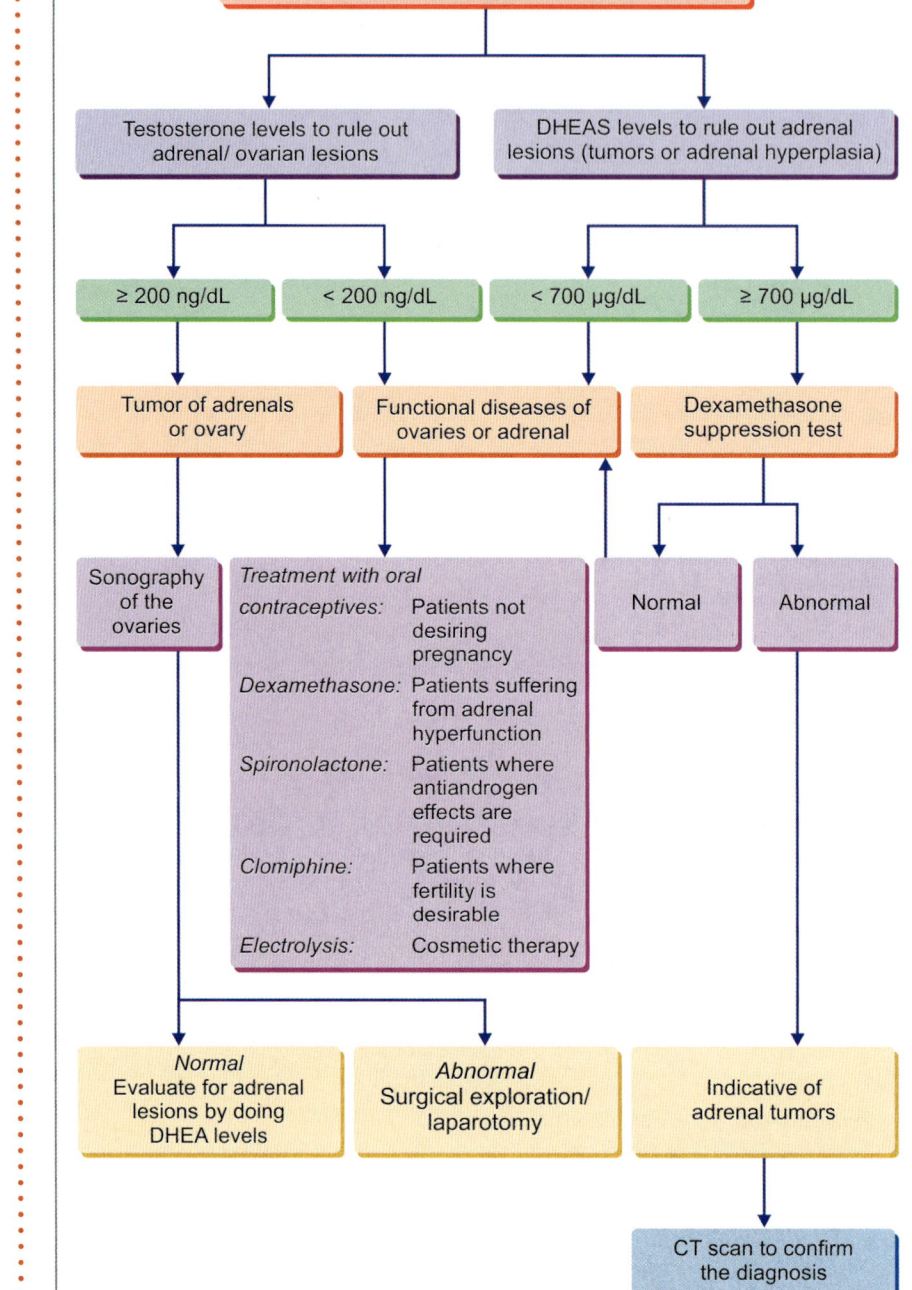

Flow Chart 40.2 Management of hirsutism

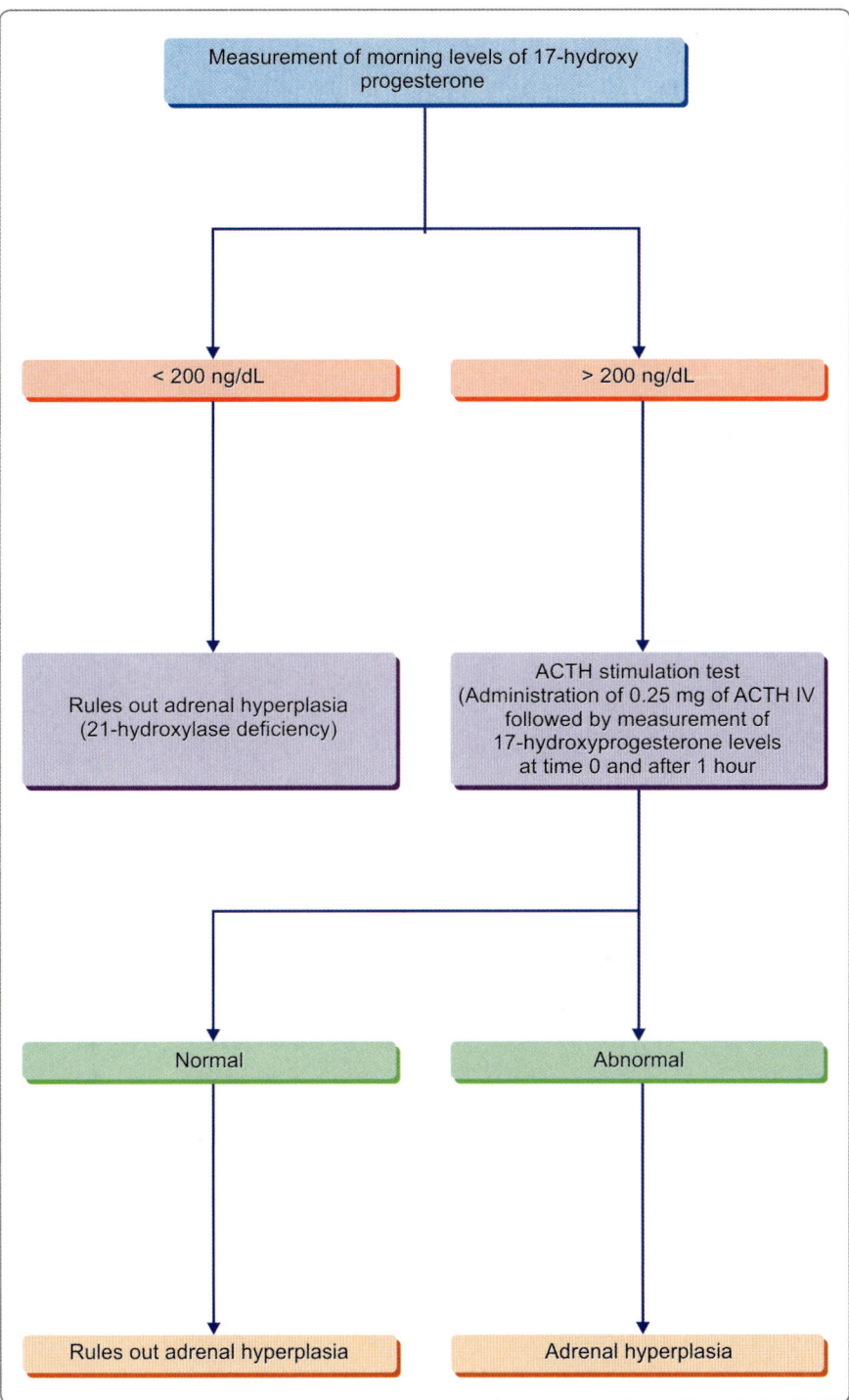

Flow Chart 40.3 Diagnosis of Congenital adrenal hyperplasia

Abbreviations

1. ABC—Airway, breathing and circulation)
2. AC—Abdominal circumference
3. ACIS—Adenocarcinoma in situ
4. ACTH—Adrenocorticotropic hormone
5. AFI—Amniotic fluid index
6. AGE—Advanced glycosylation end products
5. AFV—Amniotic fluid volume
6. AGUS—Atypical glandular cells of undetermined significance
7. APH—Antepartum hemorrhage
8. ARM—Artificial rupture of membranes
9. ASCUS—Atypical squamous cells of undetermined significance
10. ATP-III—Adult treatment panel III
11. AUB—Abnormal uterine bleeding
12. aPTT—Activated partial thromboplastin time
13. βhCG—Beta human chorionic gonadotropin
14. BP—Blood pressure
15. BPP—Biophysical profile
16. BSO—Bilateral salpingo-oophorectomy
17. CBC—Complete blood count
18. CIN—Cervical intraepithelial neoplasia
19. CPD—Cephalopelvic disproportion
20. CST—Contraction stress test
21. CTG—Cardiotocography
22. D & C—Dilatation and currettage
23. DES—Diethylstilbestrol
24. DIC—Disseminated intravascular coagulation
25. DIT—Diidothyronine
26. DFMC—Daily fetal movement count
27. DHEA—Dehydroepiandrosterone
28. DHEAS—Dehydroepiandrosterone sulphate
29. DUB—Dysfunctional uterine bleeding
30. ECV—External cephalic version
31. EFW—Expected fetal weight
32. ESR—Erythrocyte sedimentation rate
33. EP—Ectopic pregnancy
34. FEV—Forced expiratory volume
35. FHS—Fetal heart rate
36. FSH—Follick stimulating hormone
37. FT4—Free T4
38. GDM—Gestational diabetes mellitus
39. GnRH—Gonadotropin releasing hormone
40. hCG—Human chorionic gonadotropin
41. HDL—High density lipoprotein
42. hMG—Human menopausal gonadotropins
43. HPV—Human papilloma virus
44. HRT—Hormone replacement therapy
45. HSIL—High grade squamous intraepithelial lesion
46. IUCD—Intrauterine contraceptive device
47. IUD—Intrauterine death
48. IUI—Intrauterine insemination
49. IUGR—Intrauterine growth retardation
50. KFT—Kidney function test
51. LDL—Low density lipoprotein
52. LEEP—Loop electrosurgical excision procedure
53. LFT—Liver function test
54. LMWH—Low molecular weight heparin
55. LH—Luteinizing hormone
56. LSIL – Low grade squamous intraepithelial lesion

57. MAC—Multiagent chemotherapy
58. MCA—Middle cerebral artery
59. MCHC—Mean corpuscular hemoglobin concentration
60. MCV—Mean corpuscular volume
61. MIT—monoiodothyronine
62. MS—Mitral stenosis
63. NIDDM—Noninsulin-dependent diabetes mellitus
64. NST—Non stress test
65. OCP—Oral contraceptive pill
66. OHSS—Ovarian hyperstimulation syndrome
67. PAI—Plasminogen activator inhibitors
68. PBMV—Percutaneous balloon mitral valvotomy
69. PCOS—Polycystic ovarian syndrome
70. PEFR—Peak expiratory flow rate
71. PFT—Pulmonary function test
72. PGI_2—Prostacyclin
73. PI—Pulsatility index
74. PID—Pelvic inflammatory disease
75. PIH—Pregnancy-induced hypertension
76. PMS—Premenstrual syndrome
77. POG—Period of gestation
78. PPH—Postpartum haemorrhage
79. PROM—Premature rupture of membranes
80. PS—Peripheral smear
81. PSV—Peak systolic velocity
82. rFSH—Recombinant follicle stimulating hormone
83. RI—Resistance index
84. ROM—Rupture of membrane
85. ROS—Reactive oxidant species
86. S/D Ratio—Systolic/diastolic ratio
87. SIS—Saline infusion sonography
88. SLE—Systemic lupus erythematosus
89. T_3—Thyroxine
90. T_4—Triodothyronine
91. TAH—Total abdominal hysterectomy
92. TAS—Transabdominal sonography
93. TIBC—Total iron-binding capacity
94. TBG—Thyroid-binding globulin
95. TSH—Thyroid-stimulating hormone
96. TVS—Transvaginal sonography
97. TXA_2—Thromboxane A_2
98. UA—Umbilical artery
99. UAE—Uterine artery embolization
100. UFH—Unfractionated heparin
101. UGF—Urogenital fistulas
102. UFSH—Unfractionated follicle stimulating hormone
103. VBAC—Vaginal birth after cesarean
104. VCAM—Vascular cell adhesion molecule
105. VVF—Vesicovaginal fistula
106. WC—Waist circumference.